6|20

EPIC SOLITUDE

EPIC SOLITUDE

A STORY OF SURVIVAL AND A QUEST
FOR MEANING IN THE FAR NORTH

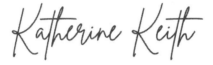

Katherine Keith

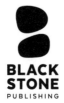

BLACK STONE
PUBLISHING

Copyright © 2020 by Katherine Keith
Published in 2020 by Blackstone Publishing
Cover and book design by Alenka Vdovič Linaschke

Some names and identifying details have been changed
to protect the privacy of individuals.

Printed in the United States of America

First edition: 2020
ISBN 978-1-5385-5704-4
Biography & Autobiography / Personal Memoirs

1 3 5 7 9 10 8 6 4 2

CIP data for this book is available
from the Library of Congress

Blackstone Publishing
31 Mistletoe Rd.
Ashland, OR 97520

www.BlackstonePublishing.com

To Amelia, whose unending faith in me assures me that I can never fail if I keep searching for that next stake.

CONTENTS

▸INTRODUCTION

We talk of communing with Nature, but 'tis with ourselves
we commune...Nature furnishes the conditions—
the solitude—and the soul furnishes the entertainment.

—JOHN BURROUGHS

It is a fall evening above the Arctic Circle in Kotzebue, Alaska. Looking up at a dark sky during a new moon, dazzling stars compete for attention while fire-red northern lights dance in universal celebration. Brought to my knees in surrender of grace, I dream of belonging. I yearn to be part of the symphony of life embodying the perfection of nature, but my song is punctuated with the dissonance of human flaws, of which there are many. Each satellite passing overhead reminds me of loved ones who came into my life before fading out into the horizon. I miss them all.

A falling star burns its way across the sky, making its mark on the Milky Way. That same burning courses its way across my heart, mandating me to tell this story. My story is not unique or heroic. It is raw truth demanding readers as participants to stand in their own authenticity. We have a choice when it comes to how real we get with ourselves and each other. While self-preservation asks us to be nondescript, the fire within demands that we be alive in the fullest sense of the word. That means being vulnerable. I trust you to handle the rawness of life in this book even though it might mean looking into your own pain without blinking.

I grew up in Minnesota in a family full of tradition and with its share of drama but never lacking in love. I sacrificed the security of my family in a gamble on the great unknown. The hunger for the wilderness of Alaska, mountains to be explored, and unexpected journeys requires constant feeding lest I starve. Our souls burn brightly to shed light on this mystery we call life.

Sure enough, life happens along the way. Over marriage, divorce, birth, and death, life gives with surprising ease and takes away with equal ambivalence. When life drags us through the mud of anger, despair, bitterness, and trauma, our tendency is to huddle up and close ourselves off in a defensive posture. We need fireworks to wake us up and open our eyes to the helping hands being offered by those around us. I wrote this book in hopes of being a bright comet to inspire others to open their heart to the possibilities around them even when it hurts the most.

"Life is suffering," states a major Buddhist precept. In eliminating our attachment to the things and people we love, we may be free from suffering. But what if those attachments give our life purpose? My life—full of attachment, full of suffering—left a mark on my soul. What we do with these scars remains our choice.

As a caterpillar spins a cocoon to become a butterfly, I seek renewal. The vast solitude of the wilderness serves as my cocoon. I enter wilderness quests such as thousand-mile dogsled races and transform each step along the way.

This book details the failures and achievements of a life that I felt compelled to live to the fullest. I may be odd in the way I find connection with the world. Not everyone likes being outdoors in Arctic storms. Not everyone needs a vision quest to uncover past memories. However, we all need the intention of healing in order to guide our lives forward. Wilderness adventures have gifted me with healing. Every life-or-death situation seems to magically parallel some deep trauma that I need to process and release. In facing real-time danger, I gain the courage and confidence to face my far scarier internal demons, the ones we all have.

The path of learning should never end, or we would become stuck in a pattern of limited growth. We have all been there: halfway up the mountain and so tempted to simply stay there, enjoying the view.

We all have the opportunity to become something greater than we have imagined for ourselves. In reading my story, I ask you to consider your own suffering and what can be created from it. What is your cocoon? I'm here to tell you it is not good enough to hang out halfway up the mountain in a bivy sack, suspended from any progress, forward or backward, waiting for an avalanche to take you away into a dark, cold abyss. Try. Take one small step forward, through the pain, suffering, grief, anger, shame, and everything else convincing you that you can't make it. Life is worth saying *yes* to.

I turned forty this year. What do I want to do now that I am over the hill? I want to keep climbing and hold the hands of others making their own journey up their mountain of suffering. You are not alone.

Part One

STARTING LINE

▶IDITAROD, MILE 777

UNALAKLEET, ALASKA | 2014

Life is either a daring adventure or nothing.

—HELEN KELLER

When it comes to cold, the crossroads of crisis and necessity is forty-five degrees Fahrenheit below zero. At twenty or even thirty degrees below zero, we can maintain our body temperature so long as we wear the proper gear. But deeper than thirty below, no gear suffices to counteract the cold—not even the four layers on my legs and feet, the six on my torso, the work gloves and two sets of hand warmers inside my musher mitts, and the wool balaclava and liner on my head, all topped off with a goofy-looking beaver-fur hat.

"I'm just a poor boy, nobody loves me," I sing out, trying to stay awake, to my dogs who march like heroes down the trail. The dogs are used to my off-key singing by now and don't seemed disturbed by my choice in music.

"Cowboy, take me away. Take me high and above to see the stars," I cry out, making up the Dixie Chicks lyrics as I go because, despite this being my favorite song, my sleep-deprived brain can't quite recall the correct words. The dogs don't seem to mind.

I am seven days and 750 miles into my first Iditarod, the thousand-mile dogsled race across Alaska. I started the race with fourteen dogs and have dropped five at the checkpoints for various reasons. Nine dogs remain with over 250 miles yet to travel.

Just as we leave Unalakleet at forty below zero, the weather service issues a winter storm warning with a high wind advisory. There is only one option: keep moving. We trek over the bare Blueberry Hills rising away from Unalakleet over the Bering Sea. I hope for snow to smooth the way but find none. Covered with sand and rocks and patches of glare ice, the climbs through the hills are long and arduous. After eighteen miles we reach the high point of this section with a steep climb. I scream out in frustration as the dogs slip around on ice while the sled sticks on sand. We cannot move. How are we supposed to do this? Inch by inch, I push the sled forward until the dogs can get off the ice. Their attitudes are positive, and the dogs march on once they get traction.

After about twenty-eight miles we reach the top of the Blueberry Hills, an 850-foot-high view with Shaktoolik visible from twelve miles away. The winds create an effect from the ground storm and combine with the sunset to give the area a glorious golden fog bank. I've traveled along enough Arctic coastline to know this fog bank will not be as heavenly to travel through as it appears. I understand how difficult traveling can be between the poor visibility, large drifts, glare ice, and low temperatures. But I don't hesitate, and we start the three-mile descent down into that fog bank at an alarming rate without the ability to stop, careening toward the ground blizzard. A forty mile per hour quartering headwind howls at us from the north, combining with the forty-below temperatures to create a dangerous chill factor of minus eighty-four degrees Fahrenheit.

In bad conditions, twelve miles is a long way to go. The wind and cold take a toll on all of us. Mile after mile, I stand on the footboards of my sled, packed with the minimum of tools and supplies we need to sustain us. My on-sled dance routine consists of kicks, squats, and any other movement I can think of to warm my extremities.

A gust of bitter wind hammers the sled, pushing it sideways off the trail. My grip tightens on the handlebar as I purse my cracked lips together to whistle to the dogs.

"Up! Up!" I yell in a scratchy voice, followed by, "Oh pirates, yes they rob us, soul light to the merchant ships." I am in my element, having the time of my life. I can sing out, wrong words and all, and there is no one within miles to care.

My team of Alaskan huskies, a cross between the Siberian husky and German shorthaired pointer, run in two lines stretching ahead of me, secured to each other and the sled with dog harnesses. These connect to a gang line, a long cable that attaches the harnesses to the sled.

"I still haven't found what I'm looking for. What I'm looking for, for, for, for … What I'm looking for," I sing out as U2 keeps me company in the solitude of this frigid night.

We leave the shelter of trees and bushes behind. The trail follows a slough into Shaktoolik. The lack of snow results in a glass ice rink on the coast. We try to navigate the glare ice, but without traction, the wind pushes the sled sideways off the trail and spins it around the team. Joy and Summit, my experienced leaders, handle the situation effectively. At last, we see the buildings of Old Shaktoolik, which indicate we are close to the checkpoint.

The dogs know straw awaits them upon arrival. A bale of straw is provided for each musher to prepare individual beds to insulate the dogs from the snow and increase their comfort. The dogs love straw, and the sight of it causes a string of barking.

"Nice day, eh?" the Shaktoolik checker says.

"Gorgeous!" I reply.

In a more serious tone, he says, "The storm will increase in intensity."

"What are you going to do?" I ask a veteran racer and admirable musher, Paige Dronby, nervous rookie that I am, "proceed into the storm or wait it out in Shaktoolik for the next couple days?" My question is leading. I'm eager to leave Shaktoolik.

"The dogs can't rest well at this checkpoint due to the lack of shelter from the wind," Paige says. "If we leave soon, we might beat the worst of the storm and make it to Koyuk, which has better shelter to rest the dogs."

I make my choice: it's time to go. I leave with two hours of rest on the dogs. I soon regret that choice.

Leaving Shaktoolik, Paige and I put on our ice cleats and walk in front of our teams, leading them across glare ice that neither human nor dog can gain traction on.

It takes a long time to leave Shaktoolik. The winds increase harder and faster than predicted. There is no beating this storm. We struggle to see the next trail marker. I stop my sled, flip it over to act as a brake, and walk in front of the dogs to locate the stake. We continue in this fashion, crawling one trail stake to the next.

Fifteen miles out, the trail changes course to head around a spit of land. This abrupt turn is unmarked because wind and other dog teams have knocked down the trail stakes. My team can't find the trail, and if the tracks are any proof, neither could many others. Heading toward land over a mile of glare ice, the dogs face a crosswind. Our plight changes from tough to very serious when the wind gusts—now over sixty miles per hour—blow my sled and the entire team sideways a hundred yards over the ice. I have little to no control over the situation. The conditions scare my leaders, and they can no longer guide the team. They can't even hear my commands over the howling wind.

We are on the ice, unable to move. We crawl around the ice in circles searching for the trail. For every foot we gain in the right direction, we lose another ten. I need to reevaluate my decision to proceed to Koyuk and create a strategy that retains the greatest number of options to get my team through the night. This is now a life-threatening situation. Paige is ahead of me; her dogs travel faster than mine. No teams will leave from Shaktoolik behind us. Thoughts of the race drop away. Time to survive.

As the reality of my predicament sinks in, I think of my daughter, Amelia, who is now in sixth grade, and drown in regret and guilt over having put myself, her only living parent, in this life-or-death situation. Wet from sweat, I lead the dogs toward land inch by inch. No help is on the way. I am alone out here.

During a momentary break in the visibility, I see a shelter cabin in the distance that could offer protection from the wind. We head toward it, and I review our choices. If we make it to the cabin, we can stay there, but only for a short time because of the limited amount of dog food. Soon we will be forced back to Shaktoolik or on to Koyuk.

I worry about getting separated from the dogs. A SPOT tracker is secured to the sled bag. When triggered, it notifies international emergency services and dispatches them to our GPS location. I detach it and put it in my pocket in case I fall off the sled. Pushing the button doesn't mean help will make it out to us, given the conditions, but it is better than nothing. I get off the sled, walk in front of the leaders, and line out the team to locate a trail stake. A wind gust pushes the sled away from me on the ice. I panic as the dogs slide farther away. I run after them. The wind pushes me with such aggression that I fall over and slam my head against the ice.

Dazed, I look around not knowing where I am. I can't see farther than a few feet in any direction. All I can do is follow the wind and hope it leads me to the dogs. My head foggy, I stumble along until I hear barking in the distance. Is that my imagination? I alter my course until I spot the team. The dogs settled on a patch of snow solid enough to allow my overturned sled to get traction and stop.

The dogs wag their tails in enthusiasm as I walk up to the leaders. I sit there for a while hugging them, seeking to convey a confidence I don't have. Between gusts of wind, I still see the form of the bluff where the shelter cabin is. I consider stopping here to get into my sled bag, seven feet long and two feet wide, with room to expand. Gear plus one dog can fit inside. In bad weather, I can fit myself and a few dogs in the bag but must leave the rest out in the wind.

I am drenched in sweat from the labor, but my body temperature drops as soon as I stop moving. My shivering signals the onset of hypothermia. We must keep going. The dogs need better protection. It is worth another try to make it to the shelter cabin before we resort to bagging it for the night.

After another hour, we make it to the bluff. I drive the team to the backside of the cabin and out of the wind. I walk inside to discover there is no wood for the stove, and it rips away any hope I had of drying out. What do I do? I can't think. I have Heet for fuel, but no snow nearby to melt for water. I provide the dogs with a snack of dry commercial dog food and frozen meat, which they inhale. The back of the cabin offers little shelter for the dogs, so I take the females and the main male leader, Summit, inside the cabin. The leaders need rest to guide us through the storm into Koyuk.

The dogs outside nestle in their protective down dog coats, lick off any ice build-up, and fall asleep, while the dogs inside enjoy the break from the gang line and settle down in corners of the shelter cabin. I lay out my sleeping bag on the wood planks of the bunk bed. I have spare dry clothes, and shivering, I strip down the layers I can and swap them out. I figured packing all this extra gear was being paranoid, but you never know when you will need it. I jump into my down bag hoping to warm up. My shivering is so violent that even Ears, whom I invite onto the sleeping bag, jumps off to go lay by her buddy, Summit.

I snack the dogs every couple of hours, hoping to keep their body temperatures up. I am out of my own food, having lost that bag on the ice. There is vacuum-sealed food, but without snow to melt in the metal box that serves as a cook pot, I can't thaw it enough to eat. I better remember this lesson well. Weak from cold and hunger, I again review my options. How can we make it another forty miles to Koyuk, let alone to Nome?

With no one else to talk to, I end up in heated discourse with the wind.

"You know, there are easier ways," I say. "Easier ways to find answers. Why don't you tell me? Let's make a deal. I am happy to negotiate." My voice echoes the words back from the ice like a mirror and hits my heart with their full weight.

Over the course of my forty years, I've weathered my share of extreme temperatures—the baking, hundred-degree heat of that left me nauseated while competing in my first Ironman triathlon, for example—as well as other stamina challenges, including solo hiking 1,100 miles of the Pacific Crest Trail. Endurance pursuits became my way of recovering from the series of traumas that sent me wandering across the country. What I was searching for, I couldn't always say. Escape, relief, distraction, answers, grace, a restoration of faith in the universe—at different times, these, more, and none.

My nomadic nature led me to Pompeii to dig through the remnants of the lost city, on rock climbing expeditions in Wyoming—the butte called Devils Tower and the outcrops in Vedauwoo—and at the granite pillars called the Needles in South Dakota's Black Hills. My spiritual nature sought the energy-field vortexes in Sedona, drummed during sun dances in New Mexico, and sweated through vision quests in Arizona. At last, my wanderings took me to the home I'd envisioned for myself at ten years old: bush Alaska, the Last Frontier.

Fifteen years after driving an ice cream truck from my childhood home of Minneapolis to Alaska to experience Arctic life, I am alone in the vast wilderness, wrapped in the solitude I craved for as long as I remember, just a sled, my dogs, and me.

The lack of response to my attempt at negotiation disappoints.

"Super," I say with a tight, flat voice looking down at my swollen, frozen fingers.

"Ears, have you figured it out yet?" I ask.

Painful emotion swells in my throat making it difficult to speak. My tired, windburned eyes look to hers, eyes that reflect pure unconditional love and adoration.

"Yeah, okay, you're right," I say. "Might as well sleep for now. The answer is down the trail somewhere."

We stay there for over twelve hours waiting for an opportunity to leave. The wind shakes the shelter cabin all night, letting up about ten o'clock the next morning. The visibility is still less than a quarter mile. The dogs are running out of food, so we need to keep moving. I hook them up, and we make our way toward Koyuk. Travel is difficult and slow. I switch out the leaders every hour to keep them fresh. Storms bring in large snowdrifts between the patches of glare ice, which takes a toll on the team. All we must do is make it to the next trail marker. Find the next stake, go after the next stake, make it to the next stake, and search for the one after that—because if I don't, this will be the last one I ever find.

▸DAD'S CABIN
GARRISON, MINNESOTA | 1988

Wilderness is not a luxury but
a necessity of the human spirit.

—EDWARD ABBEY

It is a crisp morning. Dad is an early riser and likes to drink his cup of hot coffee out on the deck watching the world around him come to life. When I stay with him, I force myself to get up early so I can steal this time alone with him. We both sit in wooden lawn chairs, facing the lake, with a book in front of us. The loons call out to each other in lonely harmony. We take our noses out of our books to appreciate the stillness.

"Whatcha reading?" Dad asks. We're both avid readers. During a recent fourth-grade field trip to the library, I stumbled across Jean Aspen's *Arctic Daughter: A Wilderness Journey*. I checked it out and brought it to my dad's cabin in northern Minnesota outside the small woodland town of Garrison. Minnesota is the Land of 10,000 Lakes, and we have almost private access to one.

I have been waiting for him to ask me about this book. In fact, I have been leaving it out on the coffee table as a hint for him to pick it up. If he reads it, I know he will take me to Alaska.

"Dad you really have to read this," I say, unable to contain my enthusiasm. "Alaska sounds amazing. It's a memoir of this daughter of a famous explorer who follows in her mother's footsteps. She and her high school sweetheart set out to build a cabin and live off the land in the Brooks Range. They eat muskrats boiled in their skins, moose guts, and even maggots. *Ew*, can you imagine, Dad? She picks maggots off their meat before it can dry into jerky."

"Wow. You enjoy reading about maggots?" Dad says with his usual humor.

"No, Dad, that's just a detail! She's tough to do that, right?"

I'd been attracted to the Far North since reading Jack London's novel *Call of the Wild*, whose canine protagonist, Buck, is sold into service as a sled dog and the Robert Service poem "The Cremation of Sam McGee" with its mentions of northern lights and midnight suns.

I idolize my dad. He's a tall guy: six feet seven. Even at ten, I fall for his same old tricks—only in *my* mind, they never get old.

Driving down a gravel road, he pretends to get his hands stuck on a coffee cup, so he can't steer.

"Dad, grab the wheel before we crash! Dad, you're gonna hit that mailbox!" My older brother, J.T., and I are in hysterics. "Dad, stop!" we scream at the same time.

All the while, he is driving with his knees, in total control.

"There's that mean old lady from the doughnut shop that J.T. stole doughnuts from!" Dad says while cruising to the local store. "You better hide."

We both do.

"I did no such thing," J.T. protests. "That was you, Dad!"

Dad holds us down on the front seat. "Oh no! That poor old lady got eaten by a dinosaur!"

J.T. and I struggle up to see what's going on. My brother is a big fan of dinosaurs. Of course, by the time we're able to look out the windows, we've missed it (see fig. 1).

Sitting around the campfire later that night, we gaze up at the Milky Way, catch fireflies in jars, and eat toasted marshmallows. Dad announces that he has a new joke to tell us. J.T. and I both groan but then clap in delight. Dad prides himself on long jokes with awful punch lines.

"Once upon a time in a land far away," he begins, "there was a mystical Valley of Thid. In this valley dwelled the race of Thids. These Thids had a very peaceful life full of meaning."

At this point, Dad describes their peaceful way of life for eight full minutes.

"The Thids had a major problem though. Every night, a crazed giant stormed down from a nearby mountain and kicked random objects all over the village. This giant even kicked Thids, including the newest baby Thids."

Dad describes the horror-filled nights of the poor Thids.

"The Council of Thids selected a diverse group to represent them and negotiate with the giant."

It takes five minutes for Dad to describe whom they chose and why.

"The final selection of a soldier, a rabbi, a mother, and a politician embarked on a great quest."

Dad talks at length about the quest.

"They found the giant. The group sat in negotiations, each presenting their argument why the giant should stop kicking Thids."

Dad can stretch out a joke. It has gone on so long that the fire is dying. I pick up a log and put it on while Dad recounts the various arguments they made.

"The Thids assumed they were making great headway as the giant sat, listening and not saying a word. The council-appointed group, now feeling very accomplished, walked down the mountainside. They assumed that silence is acquiescence. Until the giant jumped up to run down and kick everyone off the mountain.

"The rabbi was last. Sensing his impending doom, he asked, 'Why did you do that, giant? I thought we came to terms!'

"The giant pulled back his leg to kick the rabbi, but before his very large foot impacted the Thid, the giant said—" Dad chooses this moment to stop and take a sip of his Coke. I know the punch line is coming. "Where was I?"

"Dad!" we scream out.

"Oh, I know," he says, "The giant said, 'Silly rabbi, kicks are for Thids!'"

"Daaad!" J.T. and I groan in agony. "How could you do that to us?" We break out in endless giggles and eat another s'more.

The next morning, I set out on my daily hike to the nearby beaver dam to check on their progress. I pull socks up over my pants so the ticks can't climb up my legs, and I put bug spray on my socks and baseball cap. Taking off at a run, I fly through the woods. I imagine myself to be a wood elf from the great land of Shannara, in my all-time favorite fantasy book. I wander through ferns, listen to birds, search for deer, and watch for anything out of the ordinary. Beyond the beaver dam beckons the land of the unexplored, the far reaches of the woods. Venturing out there makes me feel alive and brave. I find a place to curl up with *Arctic Daughter* and listen to the trees creak as they sway in the breeze.

I camp out that night in the woods. I pretend to be a great polar explorer surviving on nothing but my wits and the meager supplies in my fanny pack: a flashlight, bug spray, a few Tootsie Rolls, and some crackers. I need little food because last week Dad took us to a local park that offered a class on edible nature. I learned which berries I could eat and what leaves make tea. I am all set. I am less than a mile from our cabin yet feel the great exhilaration that comes with walking in the vast unknown.

I pitch my tent and love the freedom to read by flashlight late into the night. Any rustling noises outside the tent walls send me into a frenzy of what-if scenarios. What will I do if a big bear comes? a hungry wild dog? a thunderstorm? a murderer looking to hide? Not knowing what I would do, I spend hours coming up with an action plan for every possibility my imagination concocts. I resume reading until falling asleep.

At dawn I pack up my tent and rush back to the cabin. I love being outside in the morning, when I can be part of that happy stirring of the natural world waking. I love being in nature alone, but I love enjoying it next to my Dad even more. Deep down, I know I will live a life of outdoor adventure. I make it back to find Dad sitting on the deck drinking a cup of coffee.

"Hey! You're back early. I thought you'd be gone all day."

I sit down right away. "Hi, Dad. I finished that Alaska book. This is totally my new plan. I will live in a self-built log cabin on a lake, own a small plane, eat caribou, have a dog team, and thrive in the Far North despite the difficulties of living in the bush. I figured it out!"

Dad smiles, knowing I will have many such plans before I am old enough to achieve one. This one is different for me though. It is the blueprint for my future. Someday, somehow, I will come to know the peace, dignity, and grace that Aspen found through her years of close connection to that unforgiving yet nurturing land.

"Then you can come up and drink coffee on *my* porch, but it would be the real thing! The Last Frontier," I say. "In Alaska. Wouldn't that be cool!"

Dad says, "Well, Katie"—he calls me by my given name instead of using one of the bizarre nicknames he usually does, so I lean in and listen—"one thing about the wilderness is that it is always with you if you look for it. It's in the sky, stars, birds, grass, and sun, whether here in Garrison, in Minneapolis, or in Alaska. If you keep that wilderness in your heart and nurture it, no matter where you are, you'll always have the real thing." Not one to be serious for long, he takes a sip of coffee and asks, "Did you see that bear last night?"

"Dad!" I say and pause. "Was there really a bear?"

And so, we go on.

▶INDIANA JONES

KAMPSVILLE, ILLINOIS | 1994

'X' never, ever, marks the spot.

—INDIANA JONES

During the summer between my sophomore and junior years, I accompany a group of thirty-four high school students from all over the US, to Kampsville, Illinois, who want to study anthropology and take part in real archaeological excavations. It is here that I receive my first trowel. What appears to be an ordinary garden tool signifies my exit from the realm of childhood fantasy and entry into a field of substantive work with solid impact. This single trowel has the power to unearth secrets from tens of thousands of years ago.

Every day I get covered in dirt, my shirt drenched in sweat, my hands covered in blisters and trowel cuts. I love every second. When I'm not digging, I spend time with a student named Josh. Besides archeology, we share a passion for the wilderness and being outdoors. The two of us settle into a routine of early morning runs along secluded roads through seven-foot-high cornfields, watching the sun rise above the mist that fans out over the Illinois Valley. Josh recounts anecdotes about rock climbing near his home in southern Illinois, where he spends weekends exploring crags along the river bluffs. I am fascinated, hooked by the notion of rock climbing—and by him.

Two days after my sixteenth birthday, Josh plans a picnic for us on a plateau in the middle of a field. From this perch where we see across miles of breakthrough bluff tops and the rolling hills that surround the banks of the Illinois River, it is easy to feel transported to an age long past, lost in the vacuum of time. Even as we look to the past, Josh and I remain conscious of the future—both the near-term deadline imposed by our last day at camp and a longer-term togetherness we hope to share.

The connection between us feels like more than teenage flirtation. That night we commit to being together after camp.

Josh says, "One day, I'll be beside you when you wake up."

With a heavy voice I say, "Somehow, we will figure it out." The challenge of living in different states overwhelms my sixteen-year-old capacity.

When the inevitable goodbye arrives, we both cry, laugh, and hug.

"We'll see each other again," I say.

Placing the bear necklace he wore for the past three years around my neck, Josh becomes serious. "The miles and borders between us will never change how much I love you. Things will change. We will too. My heart will always be for you."

Countless young sweethearts share similar expressions, but despite our youth and distance between us, Josh and I resolve to develop a future together.

▶COLD
BIWABIK, MINNESOTA | 1996

The woods are lovely, dark and deep,
But I have promises to keep,
and miles to go before I sleep,
And miles to go before I sleep.

—ROBERT FROST

My passion during high school is cross-country skiing. During Christmas break with my high school ski team, I travel to the Iron Range of northern Minnesota, I view this as an expedition, preparation for my Arctic future, offering me the chance to challenge myself, working alone in the deep cold. We will stay for a week, training on the ski loops around Giants Ridge, in Biwabik (whose name derives from the Ojibwe word for iron) in the heart of Minnesota Nordic skiing country. We have the freedom to explore forty miles of well-groomed trails, cleared twenty feet wide, that weave through the Superior National Forest. The safe trails are self-contained, so we can ski alone or with a small group if we prefer. I prefer being alone. I can go at my pace, don't have to talk or hear people talk, and can wrap myself in the stillness of the Northwoods, Minnesota winter.

After a couple of days, temperatures drop to thirty below. I am skiing the Biwabik trail, enjoying the tall pine trees surrounding me about six miles out from the lodge, when I come across a fellow team member, Amy.

She is classical skiing and feeling ill. She is freezing and still a long way from shelter. I am skate skiing, which allows me to glide over the snow as if ice skating, so I'm moving faster than she. It's four in the afternoon, and I am wrapping up my workout with about thirty minutes left to make it to the lodge before darkness falls and the kitchen closes.

I can't leave her behind, so I join her at what feels to be a crawling pace. They groom the trails with classical tracks on the side and a wide skating lane at the center, so we can ski side by side. I try to keep her going with my witty banter.

"So, this is fun, right?" I say with a half laugh.

"Seriously?" Amy says, shivering through gritted teeth.

"Isn't this everything we hope for? Adventure, companionship, and good stories to tell?"

"Yeah, not so much," Amy says. "This is a mandatory trip. Wilderness and I don't go hand in hand."

I laugh out loud thinking she is joking. "Wilderness, hah! This isn't wilderness. We're on a groomed ski trail. Good one."

Silence answers me.

Nordic ski clothes are designed to keep you warm while your body is moving. They're tight-fitting to allow movement without added bulk or restriction, and they're made of material that breathes while protecting you from the biting wind. The gloves need to be thin enough to fit the ski pole, and the ski boots are small with little insulation. This active clothing doesn't keep you warm while out on a gentle stroll, and it isn't long before I begin to feel the chill.

At this slow pace I can hear the crunching sound of my skis gliding over the diamond crystals of snow beneath the waxed surface and appreciate the hoarfrost icicles on the towering pine trees. A team of sled dogs lined out in front of me is all that is missing. The cold creeps into my bones. First my fingers hurt, and no matter how many arm circles I do, the blood doesn't reach my fingers quickly enough for them to keep any heat. My toes feel like ice blocks and are unable to move. The tip of my nose feels like a giant spider bit it. I triage the cold areas, trying to do things to warm up. I lose ground and my shivering becomes uncontrollable.

Amy and I are now in good company, freezing together.

"Fun you say?" she asks.

I try to keep up my good spirits. "Yeah, I love this. Fresh air is so invigorating. This is great for burning calories too."

It takes us about two hours to get back to the lodge, and we arrive in the dark. Being raised in northern Minnesota, I am not unaccustomed to cold. Once inside the bunkhouse, our white hands warm and turn a deep purple. Pain shoots through my extremities as I regain my body temperature. The coaches throw Amy and me in a warm shower followed by buddying us up in a sleeping bag—cozy but effective. It is the first time I recognize in a tangible, corporeal way the real dangers of severe cold.

▸DOG MUSHING 101
KOTZEBUE, ALASKA | 2018

There is no such thing as a problem without a gift for you in its hands. You seek problems because you need their gifts.

—RICHARD BACH

Let me tell you about Ears. Ears is now nine years old and the purest of companions one can find. When I am despondent, she consoles me. I think of her, and she looks up my way with her bright blue eyes with dark specks bordering her irises. Ears is an alpha female, meaning she enjoys fighting with every other gal in the yard who threatens her place in the world. The only human she wants to be with is me—pure loyalty. No dog or other human will dictate terms to her. While a serious sled dog, she plays inside with a giant green rubber ball, waiting for me to pick it up and throw it back to her. When I'm not there, she plays catch with herself (see figs. 2 and 3).

Ears has been my leader for six years and has never quit on me, even in the most difficult situations. Through blizzards, cold nights, long runs, and everything in between, Ears has been at the front looking back at me and smiling. Yes, dogs do smile. She exemplifies the true heart of a sled dog. She wants nothing more than to be leading the pack and looking out toward the next horizon with me at her side. While racing, we exhaust ourselves, but Ears has the fire within to stand up and keep us going down the trail with an enthusiasm I only hope to one day match.

Let me tell you about Summit. Summit is a regal leader through and through. He knows he is king but in a humble manner that doesn't demand submission. A beautiful, solid male with a unique blue fur coat that makes him stand out from any other dog. His upright posture and noble demeanor inform us all that we are in the presence of power and grace. Summit can see through to your soul and know what is needed without being told. All dogs are willing to follow his lead. He is serious yet loves affection and praise (see figs. 4 and 5).

Summit has led me through many hazards: blizzards, crazy-thin glare ice with sideways winds, snow up to our thighs, and overflow so deep the dogs have to swim. He is the epitome of a sled dog leader. Not only is he gorgeous and strong with a fiery willpower, but he has the intelligence to find his way along the trails and the heart to care enough to pull the musher and team to safety.

Let me tell you about Blondie. Blondie came to us from the kennel of Kelly Maixner and was three years old when I first met him. Physically, Blondie has the build of an Ethiopian marathoner. His fur is thin and light colored, and there is hardly any of it on his belly. My first thought was that this dog won't make in the Arctic (see fig. 6).

Then, I saw him run, got to know his personality, and watched in amazement as his heart proved to be five times bigger than his skinny body. This tiny dog, by himself, in single lead, would time and again lead the entire team through thousands of miles of difficult trail. He is somewhat socially awkward but leans into my legs for assurance and affection whenever I stand near him. I have never seen anything like it. Before long, Blondie became my number one leader, ever ready to give you his all.

Now, let me tell you about Rambo. Rambo is a team dog. The lead dogs aren't the only critical part of the team. Rambo was never technically a leader, as far as running at the front of the team goes, but he was the strongest of team dogs for his entire career. There never was a more resilient and capable dog than Rambo. When it is time to go, he is the first one standing. When the winds blow strong, Rambo leans into them. When all else is going wrong and the team has nothing left to guide them, Rambo stands up, barks, and pulls the team and me through with the sheer force of his will—toughest dog I have ever met (see fig. 7).

That is the thing about sled dogs. Beyond being exceptional athletes, they exemplify characteristics we aspire to. They mirror unconditional love, loyalty, determination, strength, and willpower. Beyond that of our ever-faithful house dogs, sled dogs have equally the respect and trust to go into unknown conditions. These dogs are born with an inherent love of travel and the ability to run.

There is an unparalleled camaraderie found in traveling with your closest companions, and that is exactly what you get in dog mushing races. Dog races can be categorized by distance—either as sprint, middle distance, or long distance. Sprint races, such as the Fur Rondy Open World Championship Sled Dog Races in Anchorage, are run in heats over a few days, each heat averaging about twenty-five miles. Middle-distance races span one hundred to five hundred miles and include the Kobuk 440 in Kotzebue and Kuskokwim 300 in Bethel. Long-distance races are over five hundred miles long and include the Yukon Quest, running between Whitehorse and Fairbanks, and the Iditarod Trail Sled Dog Race, which runs 1,049 miles from Anchorage to Nome. In the races, teams start out with twelve to sixteen dogs, but during training, teams can be anywhere from five to twenty-four dogs.

While considered to be Alaskan huskies, sled dogs are not a breed recognized by the American Kennel Club. Alaskan huskies weigh between forty and sixty-five pounds and are bred for speed, endurance, power, intelligence, fur, feet, attitude, among other distinguishing attributes. They are serious athletes, not pets. Affectionate sled dogs have the heart to run in camaraderie with their musher. Some sled dogs are more akin to wolves, however, and don't care for the affection of their human musher. They don't bother about adoration and snuggling. They have the soul to devour meat, pull, and run to the next adventure.

Each dog holds a unique place along the gang line. The lead dogs run out in front of the others. Their job is vital to the success of the team. Fearlessly, they find the trail and keep the team lined out true as an arrow.

The bond between musher and lead dog is trusting, deep, and pure, born of mutual respect. Swing dogs stay behind the lead dogs and help them swing the team around any turns. Wheel dogs are in the back of the team, and their role is to keep the sled lined out as it goes around tight corners.

Mushers teach sled dog leaders common commands such as "gee" (go right) and "haw" (go left). The words "up, up" or a whistle signals to the dogs that it is time to go. "Whoa" tells them to halt.

When racing long-distance, sled dogs require over 10,000 calories per day. At home, during standard training, this is closer to 2,500 calories. Whether racing or at home, each dog eats a warm meal of meat, fish, fat, and commercial dog food. Between meals, I give my dogs snacks of frozen fish, meat, or fat, depending on the nutritional needs of each. I occasionally give other supplements according to demand.

While racing, all dogs wear booties to protect their feet from rough trail. Booties prevent snow from balling up on the pads of their feet and cuts from sharp ice. They come in a variety of shapes and sizes but have the general appearance of a sock with a piece of Velcro to secure it to the foot.

All mushers have a game plan before starting a race. For example, a team may run for six hours then rest for four. Some teams travel over ten hours and take a longer break. Mushers train the team for a specific run-rest schedule to use during races.

All middle-to-long-distance races have checkpoints that store food that mushers ship out for the dogs. These checkpoints also host veterinarians and other race volunteers. When a dog becomes ill or injured on the trail, a musher carries them in the sled to the next checkpoint, where pending transport back home, the dogs are cared for by the veterinarians.

When it is time to rest, the musher secures the sled, then puts out straw beds for all the dogs and removes their booties. I remove tug lines so that only necklines attach the dogs to the gang line. The dog cooker, a portable spirit stove, melts snow for dog food and water. Meanwhile, the dogs receive a massage while I evaluate their condition. After feeding the dogs, the musher eats a precooked meal packed in a vacuum-sealed pouch. Depending on the duration of overall rest, a musher may get forty-five minutes to three hours of sleep. If the team is at a checkpoint, there is often water provided and a type of shelter to sleep in. If the team is camping outside, however, mushers often sleep in a sleeping bag atop their sleds, but a few erect tents or bivy sacks to slumber in.

Modern racing sleds are lightweight and often have aluminum or carbon fiber frames. The frame sits on aluminum runners to which removable plastic strips are attached for smooth gliding across the snow. A gang line stretches in front of the sled and translates the pulling power of the dogs from their harnesses to the sled. Padded by the manufacturers, the harnesses, fit around the dogs' shoulders and forelegs and are connected to the gang line by sections of rope called tug lines. Sleds have a minimum of two metal hooks to anchor the team for short periods so the musher can stop when required. A sled bag fits inside the frame and holds all needed gear. During a race, mandatory sled gear includes a cold-weather sleeping bag, hand ax, snowshoes, booties, dog food, and a dog cooker for melting snow and cooking dog food using Heet or methanol as fuel.

Each dog is subjected to stringent workups before being permitted to take part in a long-distance race, including an EKG test, blood work, and a physical examination. For a race, like the Iditarod, well over ten thousand routine checkpoint veterinary examinations take place by one of the dozens of volunteer veterinarians.

The top race official is the race marshal and he or she is assisted by race judges at each checkpoint. They are in place to ensure that mushers adhere to race rules and that they provide proper dog care. The trail committee will not tolerate inhumane treatment. Each checkpoint also has a checker, who records the time and number of dogs in the team upon arrival and departure from the checkpoint.

Volunteers—over 1,500 of them—are the heart of the race. They put together the trail, handle pre- and post-race banquets, care for dropped dogs, solicit donations, and take care of a myriad other details.

Mushers are a unique breed of their own. They are unsupported during the race and must have no outside help. Men and women are equal competitors on the trail. A skilled musher will have drive, experience, wilderness knowledge, swift judgment, and survival skills. These qualities matter more than brute strength and fitness.

Mushers must dress and be prepared for extreme conditions. Layering is the most effective technique. Weather can be anything from sixty degrees Fahrenheit below zero to forty above and raining. Our bodies lose up to 50 percent of their heat through the head and neck. Mushers therefore prioritize quality hats and hoods, often made with beaver, wolverine, or wolf fur.

Why do mushers push the limits of human endurance in collaboration with a team of their closest companions doing the same? The answer is indisputable: it's the dogs, the wilderness, the challenge, the beauty. And did I mention the dogs?

►KOBUK 440

KOTZEBUE, ALASKA | 2012

May your trails be crooked, winding, lonesome, dangerous, leading to the most amazing view. May your mountains rise into and above the clouds.

—EDWARD ABBEY

The Kobuk 440 race has a history of mushers taking a main traveling trail that is not part of the official race trail. Some years, the Kobuk 440 board allows use of the "cut-off." This year, they don't. I have not traveled by dogs to Noorvik and am clueless about where this cut-off trail is. Markers are sparse and knocked over. At three o'clock in the morning, on the last forty miles of trail, I follow the brightest markers I can find, including a nice big *XX* marking. They look like beacons out of nowhere calling me to them. I go along my way, happy to be on the trail. The dog team is on fire, and there is no stopping them. Every dog travels with pure grace. Their paws land in sync with each other, as if they are not even touching the ground. The leaders eat up the trail with drive and hunger to chase down mile after mile. I just keep quiet, watch in wonder, and try to stay out of their way. Our team is catching up. We will win this race.

I see two snow machines, the preferred term for snowmobiles in Alaska, coming up behind me and waving at me to stop. The race marshal gets off his machine, walks up, and tells me I am disqualified. I need to go back to the river and continue to Kotzebue, where the Kobuk 440 board will decide what to do with me. I don't understand what he is saying. I am disqualified? For what? Unlike in the Yukon, in Alaska double *X*s are a hazard marking, not a glorious sign from God to go that way. Knowing how the trails are marked in the region I am traveling would be smart.

I make a U-turn with the dogs, going back one hour to the river. The dogs' attitude plummets, and their nine-mile-per-hour speed crashes to six. I am a basket case after not sleeping for three days and working hard to perfect my first race. I crash. I cry out loud, screaming in frustration—all things you do *not* do when you have a team of dogs keyed to your attitude. Mushers don't have the luxury of breaking down. The dogs' collective attitude mirrors my mental state even when I don't say a word. They feel it. They know when I am faking it. I have to feel genuinely positive, confident, and strong, or they won't. Needless to say, I don't succeed in this tonight. We maintain our six-mile-per-hour speed back to Kotzebue, finishing in fourth place—a very important lesson learned.

According to the Iditarod race rules, before registering, you must run two or more approved 300-mile qualifying races and at least one approved 150-mile qualifying race. That's three races—unless you have run the Yukon Quest, in which case you need no other qualifiers. Many options exist, but living in Kotzebue means I both want and need to complete the Kobuk 440 twice and the Kuskokwim 300. Upon completion, the race marshal signs a form certifying my aptitude as a musher, which serves as a recommendation, a stamp of approval certifying that I won't kill myself out there. My rookie Kobuk 440 race in April 2012 is my first middle-distance dog race. I have a phenomenal team of dogs from John Baker's 2011 champion Iditarod team. They are the best canine athletes in the world—and I am the most inexperienced musher.

The Kobuk 440 is a local race starting and ending in Kotzebue, Alaska. Much of the history of the Kobuk 440 race is unwritten, but the oral history stays with the people who have lived it and the generations that came before them. The Kobuk 440 allows twelve dogs per team and goes through the northwest Alaska village checkpoints of Noorvik, Selawik, Ambler, Shungnak, Kobuk, and Kiana (see fig. 8).

I have the pleasure to run two littermates, Ocean and Ripple. Both dogs are this rare blue color and have similar builds. But that is where the resemblance stops—one is male, the other female.

Halfway through the race, I switch up leaders, thinking Ripple's spunk will get us to the next checkpoint. I experience odd issues with Ripple— she is not acting like herself. The line is loose, and she is messing around with Velvet, the other female leader. We make our way to Shungnak, and there is a photographer kneeling on the ground fifteen yards away from the trail. Ripple takes off after the photographer. We are on glare ice, and I have no way to stop the team.

I wave my hands to get the photographer's attention. Within three feet of him, I come across a patch of snow and manage to stop the team. Maybe this is normal for the dogs, what do I know? As we get on through a couple more checkpoints, I continue to have trouble with Ripple not listening. She may not be listening, but she's driving the team at a great pace, and I'm eager to keep that up. After she chases down some kids eating hot dogs on the way back through Shungnak, I remove her from lead and put Summit, her father, up front. It is only then I realize "she" is instead a "he"—Ocean has just led the team for the first time!

That mistake did not impact my race—but taking the wrong trail out of Noorvik did.

►ROCK CLIMBING

LARAMIE, WYOMING | 1997

Man cannot discover new oceans until
he has courage to lose sight of the shore.

—PROVERB

On the outside, I am full of life, passion, and vitality. I work hard for the things I want. I yearn to experience wild places, athletics, dog teams, a family, archaeology, and Josh. I want my dream life inspired by *Arctic Daughter.*

Secretly however, my inner life holds little joy, with significant pain and suffering. I have constant nightmares that are mismatched to my reality. Gory, violent, and troubling, they make little sense. By the morning, I shake off the horror and paste an energetic smile on my face. This dissonance is what eating disorders thrive on. It starts slowly at first as if to ease me into the addiction. Before long, bulimia is my only friend. When I feel hurt, it comforts me. It masks my emotional pain so I don't have to deal with it. It gives me a shelter to hide in, where I can leave life's problems behind and focus on nothing but counting calories and the scale. My wilderness nature, active lifestyle, and passion for learning seem at odds with mental illness, which can be consuming.

I have no excuse. My parents got divorced when I was four. So what? They had two new kids each with new families. That's cool. My mom's new husband is a jerk. Whatever. Many bigger problems are going on in the world. How am I so self-centered that I can't control this mental disease? I have no clue what my problem is. The nightmares continue.

My eating disorder is a secret until I am ninety-four pounds and too weak to pursue my outdoor passions with the required energy. After a month's stay at an inpatient program for my eating disorder, I head west, first to the Needles mountain peaks in Arizona and later to Devils Tower. I am seventeen years old.

Josh and I meet up for our first rock climb in Giant City State Park in Illinois, where a thick canopy of trees shelters a mossy, craggy cliff. Never one to let lack of equipment stand in his way, Josh supplies us with an old rope from his grandparents' cellar and some harnesses knotted together out of pieces of scrap cord. After anchoring the rope to a tree, he teaches me how to find footholds in my street shoes and to make my way up the rock face hanging on by my fingertips. I love the purity and minimalism when I experience my first real outdoor climb, savoring being twenty feet off the ground, trusting my partner to catch me if I fall. We are in God's playground.

Determined to learn as much as I can over the ensuing months, I progress from beginner-level sport climbs to leading traditional, multipitch climbs, high up, with views of exquisite places. Climbing offers me escape, connection, and challenge. It offers solace to the soul, making the eating disorder seem far away.

Two years later I continue to climb. You can find climbing partners just by showing up. Have your own gear, practice due diligence with the person you choose as a partner, but don't let a thing like no partner hold you back. While climbing on Devils Tower, I meet two guys who invite me to go with them to Laramie, Wyoming, to climb in Vedauwoo. I stay there for a while, working at a local bakery. Climbing fills the rest of my hours, allowing me to test my skills at a new level. If you count the doughnuts and day-old bread I take home at day's end, it is a sweet situation.

In Vedauwoo I learn to night climb. The idea flummoxes me until I understand just how much you can perceive in moonlight. I revel in the dramatic beauty of the moonlight mirrored on the surface of the rock face as I dance my line up the climb, Cat Stevens' song "Moonshadow" in my head. I sing to the poor rocks, "I'm being followed by a moonshadow, moonshadow, moonshadow. And if I ever lose my way, I won't moan, and I won't beg." Butchering a classic, I continue, "Did it take long to find me? I ask the faithful light. Did it take long to find me? Will you tell me what's right?" Once I know a basic melody, I can sing all night with gusto.

Crack climbing, where you follow a crack in the rock and use specialized climbing techniques to ascend, becomes my favorite climbing style. The cracks vary in size from those barely big enough for fingers to those so wide the entire body can fit inside. One scorching summer day in June, I lead a traditional climb on Currey's Diagonal, rated a 5.10c3 on the Yosemite Decimal System. A 5.10 climb is one that a dedicated weekend climber might attain. 5.11 remains in the realm of a hardcore climber, which I aspire to be. The last, and only, protection available along a fifteen-foot span forty feet above the ground is a tiny pine tree, around which climbers wrap webbing. I put a tiny nut in a crack with sweaty hands on nonexistent footholds, when my left foot slips. It is all over.

No, the tiny pine tree holds. It's a miracle. Since my partner has given out a lot of slack to keep from throwing me off balance, I fall at least thirty feet onto a rock outcropping below, where both my ankles hit hard before tension on the rope bounces me back up. Torn ligaments in both ankles leave me unable to walk for a couple of weeks and unable to climb for almost a year.

Rock climbing is more than an athletic challenge for me. It fosters my connections to other people and to the natural world, a salvation for my teenage self. Now I have to find alternative channels. My nomadic nature calls me back to the road, so I wander on. I leave Laramie. I am now eighteen years old, roaming the western states, living out of my car.

I drive to Arizona to explore Flagstaff and Sedona. While hiking in Sedona, a cyst on my ovary ruptures. I have to crawl back to my car, then drive to the hospital. After this scare, I go back to Minneapolis and try to save up money. I work at a climbing gym and canvass for the Sierra Club, working on the Clean Air Act.

Somehow, things go awry—again. I make bad choices. I write bad checks to get things I need. I fault on a car loan cosigned by Mom's closest friend. I don't pay my parking tickets and end up in jail overnight. I owe $8,000 on the car loan and $4,000 to my uncle for helping me get out of the legal repercussions of the bounced checks. My Buddhist practices deepen, I become a vegan, but my lifestyle doesn't seem to follow that of a monk. I become a wannabe hippie. I make and sell hemp jewelry on street corners around coffee shops, where I camp out with my dog, guitar, and long, colorful skirt, listening to Bob Dylan.

Time to find Josh and get out of the city.

▸MARRIED

SAVANNAH, GEORGIA | 1998

You gotta cry without weeping, talk without speaking
Scream without raising your voice.

—U2, "RUNNING TO STAND STILL"

Josh joined the army to become a ranger. In June 1998, Josh and I reunite after two years apart to backpack together in Canyonlands in Utah. We trek forty miles through desert terrain not unlike the Grand Canyon but older and shallower.

We sleep each night by a campfire in sleeping bags beneath the glorious stars. Each morning, we wake to a symphony of birds and the wind whispering in the canyons. Everyday reality slips from our grasp, and all we know is each other and the earth and sky around us. It's not long before we have a brilliant idea: we should get married.

We take three months to arrange our wedding in Minneapolis before planning to move to Savannah, Georgia, where Josh is stationed. Our wedding is textbook fairy-tale. Family and friends congregate in a retrofitted barn in Stillwater, Minnesota. My sisters sing a cute harmonizing version of "Edelweiss." Josh and I have a unity candle ceremony and write our own vows. Everything is brilliant, full of happiness, and I can't help but weep for joy. When my Mom gifts me with something blue, I cry. Then when Dad walks me down the aisle, I cry. For the father-daughter dance, we play "Swinging" by John Anderson, a song my Dad would sing to me as a child without end. I cry again. Josh and I dance to "What a Wonderful World" by Louis Armstrong, and the tears finally stop. Looking into his eyes, I know we will be together for all our years.

"There is no … way you can … pick me up! You will hurt your … back! Stop!" I gasp, too hysterical from laughter to construct a complete sentence. My protests pass by unnoticed as Josh sweeps me off my feet and carries me across the threshold of our glorious double-wide nestled in the wilds of Savannah. To us, this is total paradise, though I may be biased. Our first home together—ours!—Josh, me, and Aquila and Nashya, our dogs. It may not be Alaska, but it remains full of promise.

"Well?" he asks, shifting back and forth on his feet, a sheepish grin on his face. He glances at me, full charm, with his head cocked and one eye open. How can I hold my own with him?

"I love it. How did you find this place? It's perfect!" Looking around, I see possibility and a future. I will work on the house while Josh is on duty. The dogs can run around and be as crazy as they want outside, year-round.

"Hey, the universe and I are like this," Josh says, showing his crossed fingers.

"Lucky me," I say as I grab him for a long kiss. It is a kiss of reckless abandon, of not holding back, of giving everything you have and never turning back.

After a honeymoon night in our new home, we lie in bed looking out the window at the bright stars that battle for attention with the dark night.

"Can you believe we married each other?" he asks.

"Well, I had my eyes on you since I was fifteen. You had no chance," I tease.

From our first day together at the archaeological dig in Kampsville, Illinois, I knew he was my soul mate. After seeing my mom go through two divorces, it wasn't easy to trust that true love exists. I love *The Princess Bride* as much as the next gal, but fairy tales don't come true every day.

"Can you believe it was only a few months ago that we were backpacking in the Canyonlands?" I ask.

"Yeah, we should have known better than to tempt fate. I'm glad we didn't know better."

"My big plans of bouldering in Joshua Tree vanished when we met for a week in Moab. You replaced my dream of being the wild and free wanderer of my imagination with this beautiful dream of traveling the world with my true companion—the one that finishes my sentences and loves all my faults," I say, looking for confirmation.

Josh gives it. "The one who knows your deepest secrets and monsters yet is still willing to stand at your side."

"Good thing I have no skeletons in my closet."

He pulls me close and holds me as if lending me his strength.

"Whatever, I need no man's strength," I say and turn away as if waiting for Josh to console me, before jumping on top of him.

"Gotcha!" I shout out in victory, somehow forgetting he is an army ranger now and can handle my fake protest.

He wrestles me beneath him, and it feels so good to be so close. Raw strength and manliness emanate from his body, but his will controls and restrains it. He wants me and isn't afraid to show it, but he will not demand it either—only stating the facts, no neediness, no need to dominate, only desire in its truest form. I respond by being present in the situation. The only thing that matters is his hand on my waist, caressing the depths of my soul. I feel his touch on my skin, but the burn goes far deeper. It scorches away all resistance, the past inhibitions, and all fear. He is my husband now. Feeling secure and trusting the truth of his love, I can let go and be vulnerable. Our relationship remains solid and positive.

Now married for a few months, we lay in bed with the lights off. I know I will wake up happy next to Josh in forty years. We will sit on a swing porch, looking out at the sunset, with our kids and grandkids running circles around us. Josh is all I ever want. I drift off in the peaceful grace of surrender found only in the deepest sleep.

Then things begin to change.

Endless hours drift by in dark slumber before a familiar nightmare jolts me awake. Who touched me? What was that? Dark dreams of personal invasion enter my waking awareness. I cower in frightened repose.

"What's that? Who's there? Stay away! Back the fuck off!" I yell out to the shadows of the dark room. Josh leans over to hold me closer to him, but I push him away. "Get away!" I yell, not knowing where I am. "Back off!" I yell, curling into myself.

Josh tries to shake me awake, "It's me. I'm here. Wake up!" My thoughts keep me locked in a nightmare of the past that makes no sense.

"Get off of me!" I yell at Josh pushing him so hard he falls off the bed and hits his head on the nightstand. When I realize what I've done, I cry out, feeling terrible for Josh.

The nightmares don't go away. Days then weeks go by with me unable to handle his touch. Every attempt at intimacy triggers this horrific defense system that seems disproportionate to the loving physical attempt at closeness. Josh can't touch me without triggering full-on panic in me. As a married couple, this is less than ideal. Josh comes to the conclusion that it's because I am cheating on him.

"What is wrong with me?" I plead.

"Who else do you want to be with?"

"What are you talking about! *You* can't even touch me. How could I stand anyone else?"

He raises his eyebrows in skepticism.

"Josh, how can you think that!" Three months into living together, our first fight is horrible. "I don't understand why this is happening!"

His muscular body reminds me of that of an alpha gorilla. Puffing out deep breaths, stomping back and forth, shouting at me incoherently.

"I am not screwing around," I protest.

Our debate always ends with cold shoulders and bitter silence. What is wrong with me? What am I doing to him? The one man I love beyond question.

We try to adapt and keep on with our lives. I work at a bar as a waitress, and Josh is at the army base in Savannah. Our relationship continues to deteriorate.

One night after a shift, two strangers invite me to their place where a work party is in progress. Knowing Josh is out of town and not in the mood to go home to an empty house, I agree to go. The faulty logic is obvious in hindsight. I close out my till for the night and go to the address they gave me to find no party. Only two drunk guys who want me to continue serving their drinks. Twisted. Then they take out their badges. They are ATF agents on a stakeout. Shit. What did I stumble into? They question me about a coworker, his hours, habits, and personal business. Not knowing him, I have little to offer. They give me a drink and tell me not to be afraid. Is this an interrogation, stakeout, or date rape? None of those possibilities are positive. While only twenty years old, I'm not that stupid. My philosophy of "the universe will provide and protect" doesn't cover blatant ignorance. I play along with their games until I find an opportunity to push one guy over. I leap at the chance to duck by the other agent and run out the door.

Freaking out and terrified, I can't wait to get to the safety of home. I wish Josh was home. He could protect me from the ATF freaks. No hope there: he's off base for a few more days. I drive away, checking my rearview mirror constantly in case they're following me. Fear owns me. My only impulse is to get away. Instinct overrules logic, and I drive fast.

"Josh! Where are you?" I rush home as if hoping to find him.

To my surprise, he is there. Sitting with crossed arms on the hood of his cherry-red Ford truck.

Relief floods through me. Thank the gods! Josh can protect me. I am full of worry that the two guys followed me. Then I get a closer read on Josh's body language—not happy.

"Josh, what happened? How are you home early? I am so relieved to see you. You won't believe what happened! I am so glad you are home," I say, running towards him, ready to jump into his arms. He shakes his head as if I am lying about something. "What's wrong?" I ask.

"What were you doing with those guys?" he demands.

"What guys do you mean?" I ask. I receive an ice-cold glare. Assuming he means the two I am running from, "They are ATF agents looking for answers I don't have."

My explanation washes over Josh. He has his own ideas of the truth.

"What, do you think I am *lying*?" I ask. Josh demands we go into the house to talk. His jealous anger repels me, and I refuse to follow him. "What gives you the right to tell me what to do?" I demand.

Josh says, "I am your husband, and you have been cheating on me. I have all the right. I followed you into the hotel. I know you were with them."

"What are you talking about?"

He lunges close to me with his shoulders raised and muscles tensed as if ready to pounce. "I sat there at the bar all night watching you flirt with those two guys," he says.

"I don't flirt! I have to be cordial to people. It's what the owner of the bar expects. I am *never* inappropriate. I didn't treat those guys any different than I would gals. I'm being nice to get tips, so we can get money for our house repairs." My voice rises in anger and self-righteousness.

My words bounce off his stone-cold exterior, and I realize I don't recognize the man before me. We are free spirits. Wild and free soul mates. I didn't cheat on him tonight and never could. I want to go back in time to our peaceful double-wide. Why should I suffer his jealous rages? I would never hurt him.

After being married only six months, unable to handle the mutual disappointment, we split up. We find different places to live while waiting for the final divorce papers.

Josh's parents come to town and search me out. "You are a schizophrenic. If not, you have multiple personality disorder. You destroyed our son. How could you do that to him? What can you say for yourself?"

They don't stop at that. Coworkers from the gym I part-time at turn their heads as we walk into a back office. "We trusted you," his dad says. Disappointment cuts right through me. I look up to my father-in-law. His features knot up in hatred and his hard eyes corroborate my guilt over Josh and my catastrophic relationship failure.

Savannah feels so far from home. Under their scrutiny, I zone out for a moment and my mind drifts to trees. Rooted yet flexible in the wind. The Spanish moss–laden oak trees of Savannah send my imagination to a realm of archaic magic and possibility. History fills each tree with the old stories, new hopes, and wisdom. Walking through the trees of Savannah, I am taken away to a world where I dance among the birds, butterflies, and into the shining rays of the sun. The ghosts of Savannah dance with me in wild abandon, free among the trees, cobblestones, and flowers. Coming back to the present moment of reality, I hear my mother-in-law.

"Where did Josh go?" she screams at me. I have no idea what she's talking about and it must show on face. "He's AWOL. He could be dead for all you care," she hisses out through tight lips, unable to contain her disgust.

Still swept up in the peace of the imaginary Spanish moss caressing my cheek, her comment doesn't register. Numbness permeates my skin, and I feel about five feet above my body, wishing I could go farther than that. I have no defense that seems worth offering.

"I don't know where he went. I wish I did." Inside I am dying. I want to scream back at them, "Where is he? Is he safe? Why didn't he call you, his parents?! I don't know what happened. I'm sorry. I love him. I miss him. I don't know what to do. Help me find him." But the words stay stuck in my throat.

They only want to attack me, the one who destroyed the good life their son had worked so hard to build. Thinking of where their son might be scares them. Everything tells me I deserve this, that it *is* my fault, so I don't fight back. I don't want to hurt them more than they already are.

Preparing to leave, they have final words of advice for me. "Get yourself checked into a mental institution and never leave. Never speak to our son again. You are toxic. We wish he had never met you."

Knowing this is the last time I will see them, I keep my eyes glued to their retreating bodies and the last connection to Josh I will know.

"Bye, Mom and Dad. I didn't mean to fall in love with your son. I wish we could have made our dream a reality, but we failed," I whisper.

That February, humiliated and ashamed at how our marriage fell apart, I drive to Minneapolis in a beat-up car I bought and repaired on my own. As the drive takes me farther and farther from my soul mate and our shared dreams, I struggle to understand what happened and why. My dog, Aquila, an Alaskan husky and Siberian mix, is anxious on the drive back. Anytime I leave the car, he gnaws at the car's upholstery and tears it apart. I don't blame him. I feel the same way on the inside. By April 1999, less than nine months after we'd wed, Josh and I are officially divorced.

I need a new plan. Josh and I spoke about one day hiking the Appalachian Trail on the East Coast. Together, we hiked parts of the trail through the Smoky Mountains. I need to plan out my path to freedom again and to find myself after these destructive past few months.

I am a twenty-year-old divorcee. I don't want to hike the Appalachian Trail, which seems more of a group camping experience than a solo quest. I need to be out there alone. I will hike the Pacific Crest Trail (PCT) to confront my demons. When you are all alone, you have nowhere to hide from yourself. I crave that stillness after living in a city for six months. I need the PCT. I need to walk and to think of nothing but the twenty miles of trail ahead of me and the logistics of making it to the next camp.

I spend March, April, and early May hiking around the Twin Cities with my two dogs and my backpack loaded. I hike twenty miles a day through the city streets, parks, and greenways. I put on my ridiculously large pack, fill it with water bottles for weight, and then hook the dogs to a belt. I choose a destination ten miles away, walk there and back, traipsing amid office workers in business suits all over downtown Minneapolis and Saint Paul.

In preparation for the PCT, I read a book on the nutritional wonders of corn and end up purchasing a variety of corn snacks, corn pasta, and corn nuts to get me through. Everything is on a budget, and I pack my bags according to the directions in the PCT guidebook. I have little money, so there is no room for error. I sell my plasma twice a week to afford materials for the next supply box.

On May 16, 1999, I am on a Greyhound bus heading out west to the Pacific Crest Trail. Everything I need to survive this life is on my back, and I am ready to face whatever Mother Nature throws at me. Something greater than myself lies ahead, and I am about to change my life one step at a time. I have never embarked on such a journey before. This is the right action and the right time for this quest. I carry a titanium ice ax but do not understand how to use it. I will cross the Sierra Nevada even though I know snow blankets the high-altitude terrain. None of the details matter. I will figure it out as I go and hope for understanding and healing.

I need a cure. The frequency of disabling nightmares has only increased. What demons am I running from? I don't know the answer, but I am sure that this three-thousand-mile hike is the only way I will find them.

▸PACIFIC CREST TRAIL, MILE 45

SAN BERNARDINO, CALIFORNIA | 1999

"Everybody needs beauty as well as bread,
places to play in...where Nature may heal and cheer
and give strength to body and soul alike."

—JOHN MUIR

I wake up to an orchestra of birds serenading my campsite. Peering out of my lightweight tarp, I look out upon a ceiling of clouds that entice me to walk on their illusionary solidity. The sun, still waiting to come out from its morning cloud cover, makes me wonder why I am out of my sleeping bag.

"Don't rush the sun," the birds sing about the beautiful morning. Looking out onto the horizon, I realize there are few moments or events that stir the soul as much as the sun at dawn and dusk. Maybe there is happiness out there for me yet.

As I gaze at the sunrise's white warmth, I understand that, wherever I end up, I need to see the sunrise, sunset, and all the starry nights between. I am now three days on the PCT and am full of relief after finishing a good amount of uphill climbing.

The trail offers a different reality: being in complete solitude day after day. The rhythm of walking is music to my soul. There is only walking, existing, and healing. Life is cut down to the core necessities of eating, sleeping, shelter, warmth, and survival. Nature challenges us to adapt and survive.

My twenty-six-mile day is at a close, and I walk fast, anticipating a delicious dinner of corn pasta. I saunter past a waist-high sage bush when I hear the loud deep-throated growl of a mountain lion five feet away. I recall recent trail warnings about mountain lions attacking runners and cyclists. I ignored the warnings, falsely believing that I would not be running into their territory.

I pull out my ice ax for self-defense. I grip the handle, feel more prepared, and breathe out nervous fear.

I creep away, not daring to run, worried that I might cross a den. What is it doing so close to the trail? The trail switchbacks and goes ten feet under the same spot. I'd be stupid to cross that location again. I skip down and sand-slide to the next switchback with the ice ax poised in front of me. I continue for six more switchbacks, when suddenly there is a high-pitched buzz demanding my attention.

A foot in front of me, an upright rattlesnake lies in wait. Jumping back, I scream. The snake's rattling tail gives clear warning that I must alter my path. I backtrack to the trail, looking out for predators, then run down along the trail. Wanting distance between me, the rattlesnake, and the mountain lion, I push on and try to make it down to the creek before dark. After another half mile, I hear another mountain lion in the bush off the trail in front of me. Is it the same one? Is it a mate? Out of options, I run back up the trail to where I remember seeing a fellow PCT camper.

"Hey, there are mountain lions on the trails," I yell out to my unknown hiking compadre. "My name is Kat."

"Hi. I'm Sean," a voice from inside the tent hollers out. "At least we know they are here. No sneak attacks coming for us." He sounds comfortable with the situation, and my body relaxes.

"Are you cool if I camp out here with you?" I ask. "Long day," I add, not wanting to sound like a total wuss.

"Hell yeah. Safety in numbers."

I set up my lightweight tarp, wishing for a solid tent, and will hike out in the morning. It will not be a good night's sleep between two mountain lions. Blisters plague my sore feet, but Bisquick on a stick by the fire will do my heart good.

Sean comes out of his tent to check on my camping set up. "Glad I have an enclosed tent tonight and not one of those flimsy tarps," he teases.

"If you hear me scream, stay hidden," I say sarcastically. "Do you need any water?"

"Nah, I'm good. There's a source ten miles down the trail. Should make it. Thanks though. Sweet dreams."

Deciding I like Sean, I sleep better knowing at least one other human might witness me getting eaten alive tonight. But the next day there are no signs of mountain lions, and I make my way to the next watering hole. I relax in the sun and tape up the multiple massive blisters on my feet. There has to be a way to wear shoes without pain.

►PACIFIC CREST TRAIL, MILE 72

MOUNT WHITNEY, CALIFORNIA | 1999

I went to the woods because I wished to live deliberately,
to front only the essential facts of life, and see if I could
not learn what it had to teach, and not, when I came to die,
discover that I had not lived.

—HENRY DAVID THOREAU

I divert from the PCT to summit Mount Whitney, the highest mountain in the Lower 48. Only 150 permits to Inyo National Forest are issued out of the 3,000 applications per day the Forest Service receives from mid-July to mid-August. All I had to do was walk over eight hundred miles to obtain a free Whitney permit and arrive a month early. I have my work cut out for me. I hike twenty-seven miles to the base of the mountain on the first day. The hike up to the next camp is twenty miles.

A month alone in the wilderness nurtures drastic transformation. The tranquility that grows in my heart allows me to discover communion with the green song all around. My recent divorce seems far away, and I pretend it never happened. Sublime peace enters my soul, leaving a permanent mark. In my introspective state, I haven't talked with anyone for four weeks now. Spoken words only destroy the magic of the wilderness. I strive to make my soul a mirror of the raw grandeur that surrounds me. Hoping that when this pristine wilderness is no longer a part of my day-to-day life, my soul will retain the experience and exemplify the wild.

Snow and ice now cover half the trail, and I cross at least ten large snowfields at a nervy 60-degree angle or greater. The high altitude affects me, and I feel dizzy above 12,500 feet, but the climbing does not tire my legs, nor is my endurance tested. There is something quite intriguing about a methodical, laborious ascent of a mountain. It's a test of willpower, a defiance of the nightmares that plagued my sleep and destroyed the dream life I longed for with Josh. Nothing will stop me. Slow footsteps, ice ax in hand, and heavy breathing create a rhythm to help maintain control of mind, body, and spirit.

When I reach the summit at 14,492.81 feet, I earn a new high-altitude personal record. I am the highest object for thousands of miles. I gaze out over the 360-degree view at hundreds of snow-covered peaks with no trees, no grass, and no desert. I long to lose myself and play in the corridors and passes of unknown wilderness forever. Tiny birds called flickers sit on my shoulder and eat gorp crumbs from my outstretched hands. The balance in nature is highlighted. Delicate life prances about on this resolute mountain. I understand what Hudson Stuck wrote when his party, the first to summit Denali, felt "a privileged communion with the high places of the earth." It plants a seed, along with a hunger, to know more about high-altitude mountaineering. Josh would love it here.

The climb down Whitney is extraordinary, and I glissade two steep snow slopes in an invigorating descent. At the base are two big river fords, thigh-deep from cold snowmelt. The dramatic landscape changes from one vista to the next, and I yearn to experience what is beyond the horizon.

Tonight's campsite is on a large, grassy plateau with an open view of the sky bordering Guitar Lake. Mount Whitney is now over ten miles in the past. Camping at 11,600 feet the temperature is just above twenty degrees Fahrenheit.

Mother Nature is the finest artist. Her dramatic use of color stimulates every cell in existence. I stare at the evening sky and watch how the sun works its magic, changing the blue sky into a myriad fiery hues. The mountains to the east hold a deep purple haze over their uppermost peaks, engulfing the sky below it. The crescent moon rises over the sharp gray ridgeline of Mount Helen in the Mount Whitney cirque. Over Whitney hangs the infamous Sierra Wave, a lenticular cloud with a flat wavy appearance indicative of high winds. A Sierra Wave holds layer after layer of clouds, each containing a new and varied shade that changes by the second. The pink backdrop goes from peach to a brilliant deep orange, through which I can see eternity. The immense setting sphere of light produces a fiery red to offer depth to the horizon's canvas. Above, the sky turns from yellow to turquoise to midnight blue reaching out to where Venus lives to supervise and orchestrate the harmonic heavens.

The moon faces Venus and offers an invitation to come rest in its gentle cradle. The sun finishes her glorious display and lies down for the night. All is quiet. Even the winds are dying away to bring in the stillness of twilight, providing my soul complete nourishment. The sky transforms into deep midnight blue as the stars come out to light the night.

This is why I am out here. This is what I search for. Ask and you shall receive. A photograph cannot replicate the sound of a babbling brook, the taste of ice-cold mountain water, or the smell of crisp alpine air.

As I watch the sky before me, I ponder the most beautiful places I have been: the Grand Canyon during a lightning storm, rainbows coloring dismal mist in the ravines; a lonely ancient street in the heart of Pompeii as the sun sets on the red stones; the desert of Monument Valley at sunset, glorious shadows stretching for miles and miles; the desert at night with its eternal sky and a 360-degree horizon of stars touching the earth; apple orchards in the Dolomites of northern Italy that stretch from cottage to cottage, free for the picking; Savannah, Georgia, when the shadows from a bright orange moon dance over the Atlantic Ocean; a wide mountain meadow in Flagstaff, Arizona, during a meteor shower at midnight; that same meadow in autumn, when all the aspens are bright yellow, lighting the landscape with their fire. I can forever describe the world's unsurpassed beauty.

Still, this high-altitude environment remains uncharted territory. I am enraptured with untouched places. I close my eyes to recall today's hot sun and listen to the river flow through this grass-and-rock-filled meadow. I know God is here with me in every snowfield, babbling brook, mountain ridge, pass, and peak, in the flora and fauna, the dozens of marmots. I take a few deep breaths and hear the ice cracking on a nearby pool of water. A feeling comes over me that I cannot explain. My heart is overwhelmed by nature's touch. Nothing else matters. Everything fades away. That's when the tears come—tears of joy, splendor, love, and wilderness.

Despite being low on rations, I devour a bag of granola, half a cup of mashed potatoes, and a cup of powdered milk. Getting through this day is like passing a huge test of endurance, fortitude, and perseverance. I howl at the crescent moon. I am alive and loving every second.

▶ PACIFIC CREST TRAIL, MILE 830

MUIR PASS, CALIFORNIA | 1999

What we are today comes from our thoughts of yesterday,
and our present thoughts build our life of tomorrow: our life
is the creation of our mind.

—GAUTAMA BUDDHA

The next morning, back on the PCT, I wake up to climb 3,500 feet to
Muir Pass (11,955 feet), named after John Muir who called California's
Sierra Nevada mountains the "Range of Light." They represent all beautiful mountains in the world. I appear to be the first up the pass in days.
No path, no trail, not even footsteps lie ahead. I am above the snow line
by one o'clock in the afternoon. It is gorgeous, with great snow traverses
rising diagonally hundreds of feet at a time up a large slope. Looking west,
the sky is a vibrant mix of purple and green. The moon stands out as if it's
night. To the east, the sky lightens. It is as rich as a dream. I am on ancient
glaciers traversed by people of long ago. The snow is solid; the sun's heat
has not made it mushy. I summit the pass at three o'clock to find the
iconic stone hut built by the Sierra Club in 1930 and dedicated to John
Muir. They built the hut from rocks around the pass as an emergency temporary shelter for unlucky hikers. Turns out it also houses yellow-bellied
marmots that love to shriek at passersby (see fig. 9).

Despite my love of solitude, I wish Josh were here with me. He would treasure this more than existence itself. He and I should be here together making fun of the marmots scampering around Muir Hut. We would test fate by leaning into the cold, hard winds coming up over the pass to rip us of our past. Where he is right now? It has been over a year since our divorce, and his whereabouts are still unknown. I heard rumors that he went AWOL, that he has a girlfriend, that the Army stationed him in Italy. He is not my husband anymore, but I can't stop loving him. I am hiking this insane trail trying to find myself, but how can I do that without him? He made me feel whole for the first time in my life.

Tears stream down my face despite my battle to not drown in the crushing sorrow that has been by my side since driving away from Savannah. Damn it. I am on top of the world. The wind can take my pain, take my hurt, take my shame, but the wind cannot make me whole, as he once did.

Refusing to be swallowed by sorrow, I make my way down the slopes, away from the Muir Hut. The afternoon sun melts the snow. I walk through a never-ending snow swamp, postholing up to my thighs. My gaiters offer little protection against the abrasive snow, which digs into my skin. There is still no trail, only an endless blanket of snow. I don't even know if I am going in the right direction, but moving forward one slow step at a time feels like the right choice. Seven miles in pure, mushy snow with six knee-deep river fords makes my toes freeze. The landscape surrounding me is desolate, only snow and ice to keep me company. Gigantic mountain peaks watch over my suffering and don't care for me and my infinitesimal feelings of pain.

"Why! Why aren't you here with me, Josh? We should be together. I need you. I needed you to understand me. Why didn't you care? Why didn't you trust me? I loved you." Yelling my frustrations into the deep-blue sky, I hear nothing but rushing water in reply. My inexperience expects the indifferent mountains to care about my struggles. Maybe if I yell my pain out loud enough, the silence will take my burden away. In solitude our souls can't hide from distraction. My wounded soul rears up and won't be silenced.

Josh and I are young, and maybe we can chalk up the mess to youth, but in my heart, I know we lost a chance at something beautiful, brilliant, and unique to us. Standing trapped in freezing water, I cry again in loneliness, realizing that it's Father's Day. I have no phone to call home, no way to talk to Dad and hear what he is doing right now. I bet he has some smoked meat going for dinner. My younger siblings, Tom and Kelly, are probably giving him the cheesy gifts that all young kids give their dads. They are both over ten years younger than me and love being outdoors just as much as I do. I long to hear Mom's voice telling me everything will be fine. I am twenty years old and want the comfort only a mom can provide.

My body is having a rough time now. My face has blisters, my thighs are red, and my nose is peeling. My lips are burnt and blistered and host a lovely blend of pus and scar tissue. When I smile, my lips bleed. I ripped the skin on my bottom lip off. My body burns from the sun and its bright snow reflection, which etches into my eyes for six wearying hours.

My pants chafe so much I have two huge six-inch square scars on my thighs, which makes walking very interesting. I change into nylon shorts and feel better. With shorts, my gaiters, and sports bra, I look like a beat-up warrior-princess on a journey to save the planet. If only I felt like a warrior. Standing here crying, stuck in water and snow, will not get me anywhere in life.

"Is this what I did all year?" I ask the mountain peaks surrounding me. "Have I been standing still, stuck in misery, too desperate to move?"

No answer. Or rather, the answer is obvious: Time to take a step forward. Time to accept that I made mistakes and hurt people. Time to move on.

"I can't!" I scream at the top of my lungs.

The echo bounces off the snow and rock and returns to me in orchestrated harmony. This pisses me off.

"Who are you to tell me I can't? I can do anything I put my mind to!" I cry out to the snow that is trapping me in my story of helpless victimhood.

"Fuck it," I whisper with a stubbornly set jaw.

I take a few deep breaths to calm my nerves and gather my grit before taking a large step. Holding my breath, I commit to the step only to fall through once more and crack my knee on a sharp rock.

"What was that for?" I demand of the mountain, swallowing bitter tears.

I watch the snow turn red with my blood. I want to live, to dream, to love, to laugh, to soar. I no longer care what the cost. I need to believe in myself again. I hope I can be who I am. Whatever that may be.

"Give me your all. I dare you!" I shout, this time at the moon.

Resolve fills me. I don't care if I crack my knee with every step—I will keep walking. Every step forward is a step closer to my truth, my dream, my self.

"Whatever the pain, whatever the cost, that is a step I promise to keep making every day of my life," I vow aloud to the moon. Or, rather, to myself.

▸PACIFIC CREST TRAIL, MILE 850

SENDALL PASS, CALIFORNIA | 1999

With the new day comes new strength and new thoughts.

—ELEANOR ROOSEVELT

I wake up the next day feeling like a train hit me. It is tough to roll out of my sleeping bag. Blisters form on my nose and cheeks. Water drenches my shoes. I have nine miles to go before starting another climb of 3,500 feet to the 10,800-foot Sendall Pass. As I start the day's journey, I trip in snow blindness over almost every rock in front of me. This goes on until I reach the ford of Evolution Creek (see fig. 10).

This monster is sixty feet wide and chest deep with fast moving water. Things are not looking good. Moving forward is the only option. When I slip, no one can return my scream but the raging river. When I make it to the other side, no one can hear my roar of triumph but the raging river.

Onward I go, wet and humble, one more mile. Then, I begin to bawl. My tears flow faster than the river—tears of frustration, sadness, and tremendous grief. After yesterday's efforts over Muir Pass, I've been thinking about things—the choices made, the wrong actions taken, the dark nightmares of being attacked. As long as I keep hiking the nightmares stay at bay, but the memory of them persists. All Josh did was love me, yet I was unable to let him touch or even kiss me. The aftermath is hitting home hard. Does Josh miss our friendship as much as I do? I never even said goodbye. Does he look up at those same stars and wonder why? Tears of regret keep falling and will not stop. For five miles I stagger down the trail like a drunk.

I sit down to eat half of my breakfast ration hoping to quell the tears. My eyes are so burnt I can't wipe the tears away. I take out a letter from Mom who sent me a parable to read:

I'm sitting in a quiet room at an inn hidden back among the pine trees. It is just past noon in late July. I listen to the desperate sounds of a life-or-death struggle going on a few feet away.

There's a small fly burning out the last of its short life's energies to fly through the glass of the windowpane. The whining wings tell the poignant story of the fly's strategy. Try harder. But it's not working.

The frenzied effort offers no hope of survival. The struggle is part of the trap. It is impossible for the fly to try hard enough to succeed at breaking through the glass. This little insect has staked its life on reaching its goal through raw effort and determination. The doomed fly will die there on the windowsill.

A door is open ten steps away. Ten seconds of flying time and this small creature could reach the outside world it seeks. With only a fraction of the effort now being wasted, it could be free of this self-imposed trap. The breakthrough possibility is there. It would be so easy.

Why doesn't the fly try another approach, something different? How did it get so locked in on the idea that only this route and effort offers the most promise for success? What logic is there in continuing without results until death?

No doubt this approach makes sense to the fly. Sadly, it's an idea that will kill. Trying harder isn't the solution to achieving more. It may not offer any real promise for getting what you want out of life. In fact, it's a big part of the problem.

If you stake your hopes for a breakthrough on trying harder than ever, you may kill your chances for success.

Mom finishes by stating, "Darling, don't be the fly at the window. Try the door. People with open arms are on the other side of that door just waiting and wanting to help you." She lists each person in my life who cares for my well-being. She ends with, "*Let us.*"

I read it until I calm down and stop hyperventilating. Her words give me the strength to continue up Sendall Pass. After 2,500 feet of climbing, I approach a lake. Next to it is a sign that reads Sierra Coolers 18¢. What? Maybe I'm hallucinating. I look over to see a family of three: Tom and Jenny Reynolds with their sixteen-year-old son, Allen. They are the first people I have seen in two days. I stumble over and, wow, do they ever take care of me. A Sierra Cooler comprises lemonade and rum. I have two. I eat dehydrated apples and two entire burritos. More food than I have eaten in days. The Angels Reynolds and their Sierra Coolers give me courage to enjoy the remaining climb.

The next section of the trail has gorgeous hiking with bushes, shrubs, and evergreens mixed in with the snow—and lakes everywhere. The south side of the pass is quick and relaxed, the snow still hard and easy to walk on. Looking north, I am struck with nostalgia. The view below reminds me of Christmas. The trees even have snow-topped branches. With ice on the lakes, countless streams, and boulders strewn about, I find myself in an endless Flintstones-like natural playground.

I soon come up to the next obstacle: Bear Creek. This is the worst ford yet. It is late in the evening, six thirty, so the water level is high. This will not end well. Things start out okay, but within ten feet of the opposite shore, the water sweeps my feet out from under me. I fall victim to the current, slam into the water, and rush down Bear Creek. I keep the pack above the surface until I inhale too much water. The pack falls underwater, and my first thought is to hope that the plastic bag holding my journals doesn't have a hole in it.

I tie my pack to my waist and the two of us bump along the bottom of Bear Creek. My foot takes root between two rocks, forcing me to stop. The pack, however, continues past me and pulls my body under, submerging my head once more. I pull on the rope tying me to the pack to get my head above water and drag the pack back against the force of the current.

My foot twists between the rocks; it is the only thing preventing me from continuing my downstream voyage.

I lean into the current and take a deep breath, not knowing what to do. This isn't something you can prep for by hiking the streets of Minneapolis, and the situation will deteriorate if I don't think of something soon.

Looking downstream, I notice about eight feet away a tree that has fallen into the water. If I can get my foot out and take two big leaps toward the shore, I think I may be able latch onto it. I get a rope from my pack, tie one end to my wrist and the other to my ice ax. My ankle is killing me, but the pain allows me to focus on my plan. It takes three throws to wrap the ice ax around a solid branch, giving me a very mediocre amount of confidence it might hold.

As I visualize the next action, the tears from a few hours ago are all but forgotten. There is no Josh, no loss, no family sorrow, no grief, no depression. There is only this one present moment.

I am ready. I reach down to pull my ankle free. After ten seconds of squirming, my foot pops out and down the creek I go. I find what footing I can and try to leap toward the tree. I can't see it and have to guess on its direction. I take another big leap and can see I'm still two feet from my mark as I pass by the tree. No! My heart falls. Then I remember the rope. It's still anchored to the branch. It yanks my body to a halt and forces my body weight onto my wrist and ax. A long moment goes by as I wait for the ice ax to pull lose, but it holds. I creep up the rope, pushing my weight into the creek bed to take the pressure off my hands. Three feet to go, two feet to go, one foot left, and I make it. I latch onto the log but don't stop to think about it. I retrieve the ax and use it to help me crawl along the slippery log. Within a minute I am on the far shore, sprawled out, and shaking with adrenaline. I check out my pack. All my things are intact and, thanks to garbage bags, still dry.

I let my heart rate slow before exclaiming, "That was *awesome!*"

I limp on a few more miles before calling it a day.

▸PACIFIC CREST TRAIL, MILE 1,094
YOSEMITE, CALIFORNIA | 1999

Most people are on the world not in it—have no conscious sympathy or relationship to anything about them—undiffused, separate, and rigidly alone like marbles of polished stone, touching but separate.

—JOHN MUIR

I've been sick for days. My weakness is increasing. Today I wake up feeling ravenous. I fill up on oatmeal and walk. Within minutes, I throw it all up as I start down the trail. I do the best I can to maintain my fast pace and high mileage. The queasiness never leaves me. I haven't held food down in a week. What can be wrong? I figure it's the flu and will disappear in a few days. The trail is wearing on me, I can tell. I am also distressed by my financial situation. I need cash to see a doctor, but I have none.

Thinking to rest, I continue with my plan to detour into Yosemite National Park, a place that has forever been on my list of destinations. I jump on a free bus tour operated by the Park Service to bring me farther into the park.

My stomach holds out until fifteen minutes from the end of the tour. While the bus is still moving, I leap out to run to the nearest bathroom. My stomach doesn't wait, and I puke right there in Yosemite Village. I spend the next half hour on the toilet. I am humiliated.

I run into Paul, a fellow hiker who has been keeping pace with me on and off for the last few hundred miles. He offers insight into my health crisis saying, "I bet the giardia bug got you from a bad water source a ways back."

The trail out of Yosemite is at least five feet wide, the typical minimum tourist standard. It is beautiful out here—Yosemite National Park the way people should experience it, hearing the encompassing rush of the raging, ever-changing Merced River. I vow to not take the river's multifaceted demeanor for granted. It is now full of life, and sometimes you can hear it flowing through the veins it has carved out in the earth. If you listen long enough, voices ring out through the constant water chorus. Laughter and drums seem to form a backdrop for an unusual orchestra, providing the ear with delightful compositions—at first in fortissimo, shouting through to your consciousness, but as your ears meld to the Merced's song, the subtleties shine through. Its underlying melodic intricacies forever impress their gifts on the listening soul.

Truth lingers in the heart, and the heart senses the message of the river: Remain wild and free. This truth sings out beyond the canyon walls, beyond the sequoia forest, beyond the snowy mountain passes, beyond the mysterious blue of a twilight sky, beyond vibrant Venus shining bright upon the sleeping world, beyond the starry sky, and straight through to the heart of the universe, where my heart resides in peace, there to remain wild and free.

After twenty-five miles, my stomach calls it quits. I set up camp, and a short while later, Paul comes along and decides to join me. I start a fire and relax under the open sky of stars. It is Paul's birthday today, so I use toothpaste to decorate a cake for him, which I fashion out of Bisquick and Hershey bars.

"It's the thought that counts, right?" I say.

It is a dry night out, so there is no need to set up a tarp over my sleeping bag. I lie down in my bag with my backpack under my head, and as I drift off into deep dreams of ice cream, something nudges me and shuffles my bag around. I peek open one eye and see a big black bear's head hovering over my own. It is sniffing my hair and my backpack. I left something in my bag. Oh no—the toothpaste!—I forgot to tie it up in the tree with everything else.

I call out to Paul. For some reason, I am not afraid and feel no danger. I realize the bear doesn't want to hurt me but is only hoping for a midnight snack. The problem is that I need his midnight snack and can't give it up. As Paul wakes and stands up, the bear grows alarmed. It grabs my backpack in its teeth and takes off with it. I am in shock but uninjured.

"Wait, I need my pack!" I yell out to the bear. I jump up and chase after it, yelling at the top of my lungs, "That's my pack! Drop it!"

The bear stops, looks back at me, and calls my bluff. I keep screaming, stomping my feet, and waving my arms like I am having a temper tantrum. The bear drops my pack and runs off. Paul and I stand in stillness for a long while.

"What just happened?" he asks,

"No clue," I say. "Can you believe the bear dropped the pack and ran?"

"What just happened?" Paul asks again.

I laugh, and that helps to drive away the terror hovering over this in-the-moment survival scenario. As a hiker, I have been taught, "If a bear is black, fight back. If brown, stay down." There is no catch phrase for when a bear has snatched everything you own in the world from under your head while you are sleeping.

I find myself looking over my shoulder with increased frequency during the rest of the hike. I was lucky that time, but I need to be more trail-smart if I want to get through this in one piece.

A few days later, my stomach condition only deteriorates further. Things go okay until I eat. Breakfast lasts about a half hour before my stomach goes though contracting convulsions. I don't bother with lunch. The terrain has changed now from mountains to rocky canyons full of color and life. In this glaciated land, there are steep climbs with only a few passes in between and more rivers to ford. Brooks meander through the canyons, offering a haven for heinous mosquitoes.

The last six miles from Benson Pass to Benson Lake is a steep trail down, and the ground is under water or snow. I slip twice and get covered from head to toe in mud (see fig. 11).

It is hard to find the trail. I stop around five o'clock for dinner.

Weak yet starving, every bite I eat hits me hard. I can't even breathe. My stomach cramps up so bad I puke at least three times. Needing money to get to the doctor, I will have to take a break from the trail to find a job for a couple of weeks. Lake Tahoe is sixty miles away—if I can make it that far.

▸SUN DANCE

NORTHEAST ARIZONA | 1999

There are no words. Yet, the drum speaks.

I have died and am now reborn in the mother's womb.

Through Prayer I learn to pray.

Through Singing, I learn to sing.

Through Dance, I learn to dance.

Spirits voice melds to mine, singing up to the stars, and

whispering into the winds.

They have blessed me with the gift of death

so that all may heal.

There are no words. Yet, the drum is speaking.

Hóka-héy.

—JOURNAL ENTRY, JULY 14, 1999

My time on the Pacific Crest Trail ends on Independence Day after 1,100 miles of hiking. The bout of giardia leaves me so sick with vomiting and diarrhea that I can barely walk. I get off the trail at Echo Lake with plans to work for a couple weeks in Lake Tahoe and get healthy before setting out on the trail again.

Wandering the streets of Lake Tahoe amid jarring casinos and night life, I am uncomfortable in the city. I've grown accustomed to the hushed serenity of the forests with towering trees rising high above in place of these flickering lampposts. Feeling disheartened, I have no real idea of where to go. I stumble across a beach undisturbed by other vagrants and roll out my sleeping bag.

The next day, I clean myself up and put on a dress that Mom sent me. I get a job at Cowboys, a local diner. With a generous payroll advance, I find a clinic to prescribe me Flagyl and begin my road to recovery. I frequent Starbucks to drink my homeless version of an iced latte: cheap iced coffee to which I add free half-and-half along with two raw sugar packets. For the next two weeks, I work at Cowboys and explore the north and south shores of Lake Tahoe. Once I've paid back the cash advance and have $200 in my pocket, it's time to resume the PCT. Off the trail my nightmares resume at once with a fervor.

I put in my notice and agree to pull a few more days of shifts. To feed my reading habit, I stop in at a nearby bookstore hoping for instant guidance on how to eliminate these night terrors that still plague me. While perusing the Buddhism section, I stumble upon an intriguing book about vision quests. I devour the book in the store and put it back on the shelf because I don't actually have money to purchase it. But I've found my next dance. While the PCT still calls, I first have to detour on a vision quest.

Having no vehicle, I hitchhike to Mount Shasta, hearing gossip that this is a likely location to find a vision quest guide. Through happenstance and synchronicity, my travels take me through Arcata, California, down the coast and east to Arizona, and onto the Navajo reservations of northern New Mexico. Weeks of searching pay off when I find my spiritual mecca and vision quest at a sun dance ceremony.

The sun dance is a historic, cultural, and spiritual practice of Native Americans, and an ideal place for my first introduction to mescaline, the hallucinogenic substance found in the peyote cactus. I studied peyote for years, and its healing and teaching properties fascinate me. Sun dance grounds are sacred. Dancers pray for unity, peace, and healing. They suffer for the benefit of all. There are fifteen dancers, six people at the drum circle, a fire keeper, and maybe fifteen supporters. The first night of the sun dance is my twenty-first birthday.

We are on 150 acres of land provided by a gracious host named

Standing Bear. The arbor circle has an alder tree in the center around which the dancers revolve for four days—four days with no food or water, without ever leaving the circle. Women have eagle feathers piercing their arms or backs. Men have pegs piercing their chests and backs. Both tie themselves to the tree from their body piercings. At the ceremony's climax, they jump away from the alder tree, pull the pegs and nearby skin from their bodies in an act of painful personal sacrifice. The skin torn from their bodies is placed in a prayer bag and tied to the alder tree.

The lead dancer's back is pierced by two pegs to which a buffalo skull is attached. He carries the fifty-pound skull, with honor, for over nine hours. Dancers are out there for us, for their family, for their community, for the anguish of those they love and all those whom they have yet to meet. Contained in the buffalo skull is the world's pain, dragging the lead dancer down and pulling him to the ground. He blacks out at least five times. My heart weeps for his valor. He has a powerful prayer. It takes four men to yank the skull from his back causing sweet deliverance—total freedom, rebirth, a new beginning. All that grief, all the history, all our remorse and torment, all of it dissipates when the skull falls to the ground. The world is reborn.

The first night on drums is unforgettable, featuring a clear sky. Better than being in the high mountains, in the low dry desert, or over a mysterious sea. It is also the time of the Perseid meteor shower, and falling stars dominate the sky. There is a total solar eclipse, and the planets line-up, forming a rare cross. Happy birthday. My heart is pure, still, and has embodied spirit with fervor and dedication.

After gaining approval, I sit in the circle to drum and sing prayers to the spirits. The hours fly by, one song leading into the next, one drum beat to the next. Unknown words come out of my mouth from the center of my being. My human ancestry, while not Native American, sings strong. The drum beats in time with my heart and with the heart of all creation. We sing at least three thousand songs over the course of the dance. The intercessor, chief of the Native American Church, has us praying from nine o'clock in the evening to six in the morning. A group of twenty-five of us sit around the fire, praying, never leaving—no water, just peyote powder and peyote tea. We sing in sync together. Raised on the wings of spirit. Nothing exists outside the beating of the drum.

When offered peyote, I accept. I take it in hand, feel its vitality, and become used to its influence. I sing and pray with it. I plead for truth, clarity, and vision so I may understand the nightmares that separated me from Josh. As people, we perpetuate our perception of reality through the distortion of life experience. Our interpretive existence may seem real to us but this does not mean it represents the truth. Let me break through the clouds of illusion and come home to the hidden truth. By being free of these nightmares, I can better serve others. Empower me to lessen the suffering of others.

I put the peyote in my mouth. It is tangy, moist, and bittersweet. Based on the stories, I expect to become sick, but grandfather peyote is gentle with me. I am freer than I have ever been. I feel light. I breathe in the universe. Spirit oozes out of my pores. My breath reaches farther than the ocean and encompasses eternity with each inhalation. I strive to be one with the maker. The irony is that the creator is ever here. I need to pray.

Spirit takes me to a realm where matter and form are not. I feel something click. My consciousness senses what I need. Spirit scrapes the insides of my womb out with a scalpel as something toxic to eradicate. Physical discomfort and nausea wrack my torso. Blood seeps, as during my period, and persists for hours. Cutting out what is unnecessary. Powerful medicine. The world of spirit reveals unreal occurrences. I overrate sanity.

"Infinite sentient beings I vow to save. Infinite defilements I vow to abolish. Infinite dharma I vow to practice. The supreme Buddhahood I vow to accomplish." Different words, same prayer. Aho.

On the last day of the sun dance, I meet a man who calls himself a healer and offers me a massage. Feeling safe after my months of good fortune, I accept. His touch becomes inappropriate—his hands wander higher than they should—and it triggers abject panic in me. Floodgates of memory open. Flashes of sexual abuse enter my vision. I drown in a sea of revelation. Demons chase me, just as they have for over ten years. But now the demon is unmasked. I never suspected him of abusing the girl I once was. I never thought it possible. How could I hide it from myself all these years? Flashbacks from forgotten years stream through my consciousness.

In fifth grade, Mom, my stepdad Jerry, J.T., Cassie, and I travel to Disney World in an RV. We stay at the Yogi Bear Campground, and my despicable stepdad hooks up the sewer line incorrectly, creating what my brother calls "Close Encounters of the Turd Kind." His sense of humor comes from our dad.

My little sister Cindy is born and Cassie, being two, wants my mom to go back to the hospital for more. Don't think Mom supports this idea.

In sixth grade, I neglect to take the garbage out of Jerry's office right after dinner. My stepdad scolds me at length: "You are worse than worthless. You will never amount to anything."

Later that summer, as a total tomboy, I ask for a basketball hoop above our garage so I can practice for school. Jerry says, "No way. This is my house and you have no right to it." Nice guy.

Mom is busy with Cassie and Cindy. Jerry isn't very involved as a parent. I live for camping with my dad, soccer, and choir.

After years of family trauma, Jerry makes my mom choose between my brother and him. There is no real choice for Mom. They get a divorce, and Jerry kicks us out of the house. We live with friends of my mom for close to a year before we can afford to rent a place. The worst of it is that he digs up the backyard pool, sells my piano, and sells Bandit, our Dalmatian. We need police protection to collect the belongings left to us that Jerry didn't already throw away. Bad man. He demands visitation rights to see Cassie and Cindy, but they come home crying hysterically every time with their own night terrors. They would refuse to go, so we had to force them into the car. To our relief, he fled the state, not wanting to pay child support. He moved out to California where they couldn't collect on his wages.

Every time he came into my room, my mind went elsewhere. To a place of safety, my meadow of dreams. To a picture hanging on my wall that my dad gave me. A little girl, her straw hat, fresh flowers in a basket, and a simple dress. She stands in a barn looking out the window towards grassy meadows with wildflowers dotting the landscape. That's where I went. I never spoke up. Why didn't I tell anyone? I should have told my dad, my mom, my brother—anybody. They might have stopped it. Guilt. It's all my fault.

The actions of this disgusting so-called man started a pattern in my life that has continued to this day. Impacting everything from sports, school, work, archeology, college, Josh, and on and on. The bulimia, the depression, the searching, the struggles—all of it was to hide from those memories. I want to turn it away, to rampage in fear and disgust. My body shivers in horror, shock, disbelief, and guilt.

▶INIPI

NORTHEAST ARIZONA | 1999

Three things cannot be long hidden:
the sun, the moon, and the truth.

—GAUTAMA BUDDHA

The morning after that fateful and ill-conceived massage, the sun dance ends. I seek out a co-op reputed to have an Inipi—the Lakota term for a sweat lodge. But the word means far more to the Lakota than this: it means "to live again." To live anew, we have to discard what is no longer a part of our greatest good. A vision quest seeker enters an Inipi to let a part of themselves be shed, or die, so they may be reborn and live again.

A local co-op farm, doubling as a hippie commune, maintains an Inipi. Co-op people live there in exchange for harvesting vegetables. A co-op worker offers to give me a tour of the facility's greenhouse, nursery beds, and vegetable gardens. The co-op delivers fresh boxes to locals with a subscription. Our tour ends at a small, round dome lodge, tall enough for one individual, at the center of a clearing. Along the tour, I express my interest in the Inipi and completing a vision quest, and the co-op staff are glad to accommodate my request.

I enter the Inipi, this small cavity of mother earth, with no food, water, or people.

"I will be back in thirty hours," the guide says. "Do *not* leave the Inipi." I am mortified. "How do I use the bathroom?" I ask.

He shakes his head as if wondering how I could ask such thing when the vast Spirit—capital S—is all around me.

I laugh in nervous anticipation, hoping that the great Spirit doesn't perceive my fear or become offended by my primary needs. Just prayer— prayer for two nights and three days. I perform an essential clearing ritual with sage, sweet grass, and cedar to honor the four directions, as I learned from the sun dance. Then I sit on a blanket in complete darkness and wait to see what the Spirit will bring.

My body is numb and my brain is distant from the recent revelations. For years, I've been trying to figure out my self-destructive tendencies— the recklessness, the eating disorder, the drinking, the hitchhiking— and have been unable to insulate those I love from their impacts. Such behaviors have no place in the life I want. I am grateful for the truth yet plagued by it. In embracing my past, I might let it go. Let the winds take responsibility, guilt, and shame back to their rightful owner.

With infinite patience, I wait in stillness for at least five full minutes. Then I go berserk. I have places to go and things I want to do. Am I supposed to squat here for thirty more hours doing nothing? Time to get up. I'm hungry and thirsty. Time to get up! I neglected to call my mom. She will worry about me. *Time to get up!* I am eight minutes into the thirty hours. My legs go numb. It's cold—brrr. Is that a spider? Do I have to pee? Is that my bladder? Should I sneak out now before the thirty-hour period really begins? But then I would have to redo the previous eight minutes. Maybe I am being watched and someone will tattle on me if I slip out to use the bathroom. Will my guide shoot me with a BB gun? Am I expected to summon the glorious Spirit in the sky and ask what to do?

After a few hours, my mind resigns itself to the fact we are doing this. I will remain here and not leave until I receive answers. My mind stops fighting me. My body, mind, and spirit work together to sort out where my life is going and what my purpose is.

Needing clarity, I shout out as if delivering an invocation: "Please help me. Please help me get through this. Please help me understand what's happening. Please help me have courage. Please help me know what to do with this outrage. Please let me see and recognize the truth of what transpired. Please don't hide from me as protection, because I know lying to ourselves about the past isn't any form of security but serves to cripple us. Please grant me wisdom on how this has influenced me. Please give me understanding on how I can assimilate this into my life moving forward and not hold back anymore."

My pleading goes on without answer. I stretch out on the cool, dark dirt floor and fall asleep. I feel insects crawling up my legs and hear noises of life outside the Inipi going on despite my misery. I continue to lie in the tranquility of the divine womb, feeling compassion and pure love. The walls around me mirror the hug of a great-grandmother, and wrapped in the embrace of this beautiful Inipi, my hunger for answers gives way to grace and peace. I might not have all the answers I want, and I might not understand the reasons; still, I feel gently and patiently at peace with things.

I sit in silent prayer, meditate, and ask for help. The urgency and desperation have lessened, and I now trust in the Spirit's compassion for me. When I most need it, help will arrive. I am not alone in this fight anymore. With dreams come resolve. This abuse occurred, and now I have a choice about how I want to react. Do I want to be full of drama about it, or do I want to use it for self-compassion and understanding, to use it as fuel for my next actions in life?

My resolve steels itself in quiet focus: "Yes, all of those things—just no drama."

The horror turns down a notch. And as the hours tick by, something removes it altogether, and the disgust, so I can think about the events with detachment, as if they were scenes from a movie, without having a panic attack, without triggering further flashbacks of a living nightmare. In the Inipi, I sail through stars in a deep sky. I am free.

Leaving the Inipi thirty hours after I entered, I walk into the warm daylight like a phoenix rising from the ashes. The warm embrace that I felt inside walks out with me, as if holding my hand, signaling that we are in this together, that is the purpose of going on a vision quest. We are not all so lucky as to walk away more empowered than when we came in, but we all gain insight. My vision quest is a success. I stay removed and insulated from the raw memories while having full access to the details of what happened. As long as I stand in my authenticity and power, my sanity won't get ripped to shreds while integrating these truths into my life.

I discover a tranquil peace. I have lifted the responsibility of my stepfather's actions from my shoulders and placed it back on his. The vision quest has encouraged me to come to terms with the new information. I hope that my release can heal him, maybe relieve him of some of his karma, set him free. The more that free people roam the free world, the more tomorrow's children will be free. Ending the cycle starts here.

On my way back from the sun dance, I hitch a ride twenty miles off the freeway to Lake Havasu. Once there, I look to an orchestrated sky, its colors intensified by thick rays of sunlight falling on the earth. I run into the lake. One minute later, I glance across it to see a magnificent green barrier of wind and rain—no big deal. Ten seconds later, it is halfway across Lake Havasu and rushing toward me. I am a tad uneasy with the radical shift in weather. This enormous wall soon engulfs the beach, assailing me with seventy-mile-per-hour winds, hail, fury, and raw power. What is the logical thing to do at this point? Enjoy it. I attempt to stand with arms upraised screaming in defiance, letting loose my pent-up fury over events I have little memory of. My past still haunts me, but I try to forgive myself for those I have hurt and start over. I stare down the storm.

"I am no longer a victim!" I yell out as lightning strikes all around me. "I dare you to mess with me!"

The storm knocks trees over and produces four-foot white-capped waves in a previously calm bay. The seagulls negotiate the unpredictable gusts. The temperature variations in both the water and air are dramatic. Looking west through the shadowy green haze, the fiery red sun sets over the distant horizon. I remain untouched. The full moon sits high above the chaos, resting in the deep-blue evening sky, watching the world pass by.

I am full of confusion, but it is time to mend open wounds, resolve family quarrels, and connect with those I love—time to go home. I have a one-way ticket to Minneapolis. The PCT will have to wait. I must keep one foot in the world of Spirit and one in physical reality—breathe, wash dishes, see my family with smiles on their faces and tears in their eyes. That matters on this planet. You can experience far-out things in far-out places, but nothing carries as much pleasure as being with the ones you love.

▶FALLING

MINNEAPOLIS, MINNESOTA | 2000

Life has become eternal in a second.
Enfolding petal by petal the vast
wonder of existence.
Slowing down, moment by moment.

—JOURNAL ENTRY, JULY 14, 1999

Coming home jars my senses more than I expect. I experienced a major shift on the trail, while the world didn't change. I pretend that all is fine, not wanting to disrupt my family. Thus, I am not authentic. I am not standing strong in my power. I try to fit in with a normal job, ordinary routines, and regular social life. But I soon realize that I am not normal. My spirit craves the wilderness, and my heart is confused over how to integrate the memories. I do this poorly. A vision quest holds little value if you don't follow the path laid out by it.

Flashbacks fill my vision with disorienting, horror-filled nightmares. My eating disorder returns, and I lose thirty-five pounds. Then the self-harm begins. Cutting starts at night, when I sleep. I wake up with blood oozing from my upper thighs. A razor blade lies on the floor. With extreme stress, I cut during the day. I attempt to relieve emotional pain by shifting my focus to physical pain. Cutting reduces the flashbacks and intrusive images. I bleed out the memories as if being purified from a plague. Anything to stop the mental replay. The blade manifests the suppressed inner pain and releases the internal pressure. I control my pain, but this control is illusory. I am stuck in an addictive cycle—one in which I am both the victim and the perpetrator, as well as the devoted healer taking care of my wounds. Shallow slices don't mirror my inner agony. Damage escalates, deep red slits drip red onto white tile floors, as cuts deepen, requiring stitches.

Dreams of enlightenment fade away. My soul is as cold as the lonely winter weather. Days are a blur of drunken writing at bars, donating plasma, exercising for hours, and being proud of every single pound I lose. I end up downtown alone at night searching for a couch on which to crash. This pattern continues through Christmas with frequent deep cuts. I fade in and out of life—a dark shadow surviving a moonless night. Please end this pain.

An empty studio off Grand Avenue in Saint Paul becomes available for rent. I start bartending school, hoping to find work with cash tips. This lands me a job at the Hilton Hotel's New Year's Eve party. The world parties like its 1999, literally. In the early hours of the new millennium, I ride home on a dimly lit bus. In a cheap, frayed line notebook, I write out my wounds and nurture my battle scars. I'm running blind with a furious pace—racing ahead, afraid of looking over my shoulder, fleeing society's rules, desperate to escape the deadly game of life. Tomorrow is far away when my feet won't take another step, stuck in the quicksand of the past.

Like a ball and chain, memories bind me in a prison of my own making. Trapped by branded memories. No fairy dust can save my soul. I look at my feverish writing.

> My dreams are empty.
> All hope is gone.
>
> Happiness is an idle term
> For some sap who just can't see the truth.
>
> The bus rolls on to another place,
> where life goes on at a different pace.

Yet it is the same old story with a different beat
—yearning for that which we just can't keep.

Thinking the worst is over
Its return catches me off guard.
Creating more damage than before.

I don't even recognize myself. In the past I could liken my mind to an idealistic, passionate tree hugger who never gives up in a fight. Deep down, this is not a world I want be a part of. Nothing matters anymore. I am lost. There's nothing left to fight for. This world is a fucked-up place. Fucked-up people, get fucked up, and fucked over. There is no point to be here. Kill me, please. I scribble out a letter to my sisters, who don't deserve to suffer from my actions.

Dear Cassie and Cindy,

I never expected to write this letter. I wish I had the strength to stay alive. Such is not the case. My love for you encouraged me to cling to my small thread of life. It hurts knowing what you will endure because of my selfish act. I'm so sorry for any sadness I caused. I've held on for months so you would not weep at my departure. My decision will forever affect you. I never expect you to understand my decision, and I hope you are never in a place where you do. You will be angry at me. You have every right to be.

Please keep me alive in your memories of the happy times. The smiles, laughter, coffee shops, bagels, and other cherished times. Never forget what once was. Be proud of everything you do. Be proud of who you are. Take care of yourselves and each other.

You girls are precious and deserve the world. You mean more than anything. I love you so much.

Your big sister

Writing this letter births my desperation. The damage my selfish actions will cause becomes tangible. Am I willing to let those I love suffer?

I need help. The vision quest from so long ago taught me that help is there when I ask for it. Time to ask.

"Universe?" I whisper. "Please show me the way forward. I need confirmation I should stay alive."

Realizing I need to be more specific, I try, "Universe, you have two days to prove the value of existence." Not being in a place to make demands. I follow this up with, "Please?"—a cross between a question, a statement, and begging.

If I don't find it, I'm out of here. I rip the letter out of the notebook and put it in my jacket pocket. The clock is ticking.

The next morning, flashbacks of abuse again leave me hallucinating and suicidal. I leave home at four thirty in the morning to sit in zazen at the Clouds in Water Zen Center, seeking through stillness answers to my desperate questions. By fortunate happenstance, the doshi, Judith Ragir, is there, offering individual sessions.

Judith instructs, "Ask the question burning in your heart. Keep it as succinct as possible."

I look through tear-brimmed eyes at my most profound teacher and ask, "How can a person find the will or courage to stay alive? Why even struggle?" I feel awful putting her on the spot like that, but I need to know.

"When I first practiced sitting, I was in a very difficult spot," Judith says. "I remember noticing my breath for the first time in years, watching the morning come alive, and the birds singing. As I sat more, I noticed life as something larger than my small self and could tap into that. My twenties were tumultuous, and it wasn't until my forties that I connected with my past and came to terms with it." After a period of silence, Judith looks at me with a solid, steely strength giving no room to misinterpret her understanding of my situation. "Do not kill yourself in your twenties, because things will change, and you want to be there when it happens."

"Is it worth it to live?" I ask.

Judith throws her arms up in the air and shouts at the top of her lungs, "*Yes!*"

That *yes* reverberates in my heart. Is this the answer I've been seeking?

Judith finishes by saying, "Remember, little things create our heaven in the present on earth."

After zazen is over, I go to the coffeehouse downstairs and order hot genmaicha tea. I take out my journal to sort through my turmoil via haiku.

Dark clouds hide
Sun's light.
Life has ended.

New moon dawns a cloak of invisibility.
Yet, is still the same moon.

Full moon sheds a cloak of invisibility.
Yet, is still the same moon.

Stars lose their shine in the brightness of day.
Yet, sparkle at night to light our way.

The universe answered my question. Stay alive and live.

I now need to hold up my end of the bargain. Knowing I want to live, I face an overwhelming mountain I must climb to heal. Tired and lost, I lack the strength to fight the impulse to hurt myself. Part of me fights to get better while the other sabotages my good intentions.

In a make-or-break moment, I call a friend, Katie Nordahl. She takes me to a hospital where stone-faced doctors stitch up the cuts on my arms and legs, then admit me for attempted suicide.

The next day, I am alive. Staring out the window at the frozen Mississippi River, the stillness of bare trees and cold snow mirror my dead gaze. This is the same hospital where I was admitted four years earlier, rail thin, in the throes of an eating disorder, and once again I observe the wonders beyond the glass in a detached, clinical manner.

I speak to the crows outside, "Nothing matters. The snow melts, river runs, clouds vaporize, and crow flies. Nothing matters."

I spend a month and a half in the hospital, taking one baby step forward then sliding back a mile. My family feels helpless, and I'm sure it is very painful for them to watch me go through this. Katie continues to check up on me. Her care, focus, and determination give me strength. Her listening gives me a release. To hear of her hopes and dreams helps me to see there is a future. Some of us may find happiness. It is possible. Katie wants something out of life and will refuse anything short of her demands.

The hospital feels like a haven, but it transforms into an isolated jail. It helps me get out of crisis, but I know that long-term healing and behavioral change is on me. Day programs and therapies offer counseling and coping strategies. For me, this approach is not effective. It serves only to wrap me up in my head and my problems. After five weeks, I am ready for discharge, prepared or not. Months of struggling to regain balance are ahead, and I know I must break out of this cycle of antipsychotics, antidepressants, and alcohol. I need to save my life *my* way for this to work. Time to search out wilderness.

▸SOUL REPAIR

MINNEAPOLIS, MINNESOTA | 2000

Here is a test to find whether your mission on earth is
finished: If you're alive, it isn't.

—RICHARD BACH

I find an ad in the paper for a local shaman who does soul retrievals. I am intrigued and am self-diagnosed as needing one. I need answers. I walk up to his door in Uptown, knock, and find Timothy Cope.

"Hi, Timothy?" I ask. "Can you help me? Your ad mentions talking to my spirit helpers and that you can help me find my power animal. I need that right now. I'm feeling lost. I'm throwing my future away. I'm leaving on a road trip to find myself. Can you help me?" I say in one breath out of nervousness and anticipation. Can he help me figure this all out?

"Come on in. We've been waiting for you," he says.

I walk into his basement filled with the smell of sage and sweet grass. He sits me down on the pillow, picks up his drum, and sings at the top of his lungs. I open my eyes wide and wonder about the neighbor kids on their bikes right outside his window. Don't they call the cops? This is his house, and I stop worrying as he pays homage to the four directions, the upper world, and the lower world—at least that is what I think he is doing. I am desperate for answers and help.

"Why are you here?" Timothy asks.

"I don't know what's wrong with me. I had everything right in my life. I was on varsity teams, getting straight As at the top of my class, married to my high school sweetheart, and heading fast toward the life of my dreams. I am imploding. Divorced. Living a waking nightmare. I did a vision quest, ate peyote, and thought I had it all sorted out. Things are being ripped away faster than I can hold them together. I want to be better than this. I can provide more details if you need."

"None are needed."

Timothy drums and sings again as I sink into the calm, deep place I find when meditating at the zazen center. Assisted through his drumming, I sink deeper, to a source within myself. I want to learn more. I have felt these drums calling throughout my life. Through the morning's work, Timothy connects me with a power animal to support me on the journey ahead. He brought back a piece of my soul that, in his words, presents itself as a young girl in an Easter bonnet with a flower bouquet—the same girl in the picture hanging on my wall. Standing in a barn, she wears a straw hat and a simple dress. We picked flowers together rather than live through the reality of what was happening in my bedroom. As this part of my soul returns, a wave of grief consumes me in pure, overwhelming loss and horror. It takes a long time before I can open my eyes and take a deep breath.

"How did you do that?" I ask.

"You are on a journey. Not all journeys are smooth, but they all are rewarding. May the spirits be with you." He opens the door and sends me on my way.

Soul intact, armed with a power animal, I am ready to embark on another solo wilderness adventure. Nature is a cure for self-absorbed thinking, depression, and a life circling the drain. Being outside, without external influence, frees me up to be myself and find clarity. Here we go. Alaska or bust.

▶KUSKOKWIM 300

BETHEL, ALASKA | 2013

The spirit sled dogs have is both intriguing and mesmerizing. To hear the rhythm of their steps and see the purpose in their drive is to witness an animal in complete balance in its world, made more so by the pack like unity of the team.

—BRUCE LEE, MUSHER

The second Iditarod qualifying race begins in January 2013. I prepare for the Kuskokwim 300 all fall and winter. I exit the plane in Bethel and receive a great bear hug by our host, Mike Shantz.

I hear a loud voice over the small and crowded airport. "Welcome home!" He means it as well, "Steaks are on the grill, potatoes in the oven, gin and tonics waiting to be poured."

After a couple of days of solid preparation, logistics, and travel, this is music to my ears. We grab the gear to enjoy the promised hospitality.

Before the start of the race, a few mushers visit with attorney and musher, Myron Angstman, born in Minnesota and now practicing law in Bethel. Myron, always a reliable source of trail information, invites us for a hot cup of French press coffee.

"Myron, what are we getting into here?" I ask, taking a seat by the cozy woodstove.

He crosses his arms and leans back into his milled-log counter and blows out a long sigh. "I could tell you, but it will probably change tomorrow."

I am overwhelmed, full of uncertainty, and hoping for more. "Come on. Is there anything you can tell a rookie?"

Myron grins and raises his left hand to count off trail conditions: "I would expect glare ice, snow, water, crushed ice, high winds, bitter cold, dirt, gravel, and rain—then you won't be disappointed."

I slump my shoulders, realizing I am in over my head.

Three days later, I leave Bethel wearing bib 2, the lowest number issued to racers, which allows me to run first on the trail with a start time three hours in advance of the next musher. The Kuskokwim 300, or K300, is a twelve-dog race that goes through the checkpoints of Tuluksak, Kalskag, Aniak, and back again. It is spectacular to be on a dog team watching the K300 fireworks go off over Bethel. This trail will not be easy. The race committee went on an overland route due to dangerous river-ice conditions. Two days ago the trail had snow cover which promised a smooth ride. Forty-degree temperatures and rain washed away the snow and left bare tundra, glare ice, and water. The first leg to Tuluksak is fast, since the dogs are excited and full of energy. We cross glare ice ponds and standing bodies of frozen water. The most dangerous ice is smooth with a fresh shine of water on top. Dogs get no traction on this, and neither does the sled. Crossing these lakes becomes a circus as the dogs, trying to cling to the ice, end up sprawled out, knocking over other dogs like bowling pins. The sled slides back and forth perpendicular to the team, allowing any bump in the ice to tip the sled over. The ice-skating rinks continue for dozens of miles. How much more can the dogs take?

In one disastrous incident, my big wheel dog, Deuce, slips on the ice, causing him to tighten up, then slide backward. The sled becomes unstable and, along with me, tips over in front of Deuce. We slide along the ice, Deuce, my sled, and me. The snow hook rips into my pants, my left leg is under the sled, and I worry about how to get out of this jam. Being dragged by the sled often seems to last a long time, but it all takes place in less than ten seconds. I free my leg, right the sled, and get poor Deuce back on his feet to attack the next ice rink one hundred yards ahead. On and on.

At Tuluksak we cut down to the Kuskokwim River and head north to Lower Kalskag, fifty miles away. The temperature that night is above freezing. Rain creates standing pools of water on the ice, along with slush. The trail is barely visible under knee-deep water. Snow mixes with falling rain making it difficult to see where the next trail markers are. Arriving in Kalskag, the dogs eat well and I get myself sorted out.

"Maybe we should take a vote on this becoming the Kuskokwim *200*," fellow musher Rohn Buser jokes.

Before crawling into the sleeping bag, I take off my boots. There's an inch of water in each. I made the mistake of not putting garbage bags in them to help protect my feet from water. While they are warm now, this would be a scary situation were the temperature to drop. I try to dry them out and find a new pair of socks.

Scared and full of dread about the trail ahead, I watch other mushers getting prepared and realize the race must go on. I harbor a small hope that the race officials will stall the race pending better conditions. But this race is the real deal and not for pansy mushers. I buck up, get dressed for more water, go out to feed the dogs, put their booties on, and head upriver toward Aniak.

I have trouble again with Deuce. He is a very large dog, close to seventy pounds, with black hair. With thirty more miles to go, I put him in the sled to prevent him from overheating. The other dogs have to carry Deuce through the bare tundra, slushy snow, and water. The heavier the sled, the greater the drag, and soon other dogs become tired in the heat. Having Deuce in the sled near the top creates a sled that can't steer, and it keeps plowing and falling into the snowbanks. I repack the sled so that Deuce is as low as possible. This change makes things better but it eats into our time. We lose a couple of hours on this run, and I realize that the team will not finish in the time I planned.

Looking forward to two hours' rest in Aniak, I hope it will energize the dogs. I have the Aniak vet examine Deuce to make sure he isn't sick. Deuce gets out of the sled, happy, refreshed, and eating well—figures. One day, Deuce will be a great dog. He needs more confidence and experience. Me too. Leaving Aniak, I worry about finishing. What do I do? Call Mom.

With hopes of some cell phone connectivity, I call out, "Mom? Can you hear me?"

The breath I hold escapes me as I hear her reply, "Yeah, honey. Hi."

In controlled, short, shallow breaths, clenching back tears of fatigue and frustration, I say, "Mom? How are you doing?"

"Fine. How are *you* doing is the real question."

"Umm … well … I'm fine too." This is how our typical Minnesotan conversations go. "*Up!*" I shout to the dogs to keep them from slowing down while I am distracted on the phone.

"Okay, the 'fines' are out of the way. How are you really doing?" Mom asks.

Ordinarily, I can bluff my way through Mom conversations, but after significant sleep deprivation, I lack my usual finesse. Tears come—inconvenient, given the conditions.

"Mom, I do not understand why I am out here—*Up! Up!*—I mean, why the heck do people run this race? I don't get it. It's horrible! Why did I sign up for this?—*Up! Up!*—I will never race again. We will be in last place. The dogs hate me by now—*Haw!*"

The trail is splitting up ahead. "*Haw!*" I call out again, directing the dogs' next move to the left.

"Katie, you are always so hard on yourself," Mom says. "I'm sure it's not that bad. You are doing a great job."

"What? Mom, I can't even stand, and I doubt we'll even finish this race—*Up! Up!*—This is my last time racing dogs. We won't even finish."

Tears continue to stream down my checks as I whistle to the dogs in shallow encouragement.

"Good dogs. Way to go," I say. "Mom, how do we finish? I want to do so well, but I'm just a great big disappointment."

A long sigh comes over the phone. I can even feel her eyes rolling as she has likely heard this before.

She tries a different tactic: "Why not just enjoy being outside? You dream of being outside, in solitude, with the dogs. I know you like to compete, but the pressure makes it so you can't have fun. Just let that go and savor the adventure."

We've had this conversation a few times before. "Competition *is* awesome" I say, voice rising, waving my arms in the air to make my point to the tundra shrubs, almost forgetting I have a sled to hang on to. "*Up! Up!*"

"Sounds like you are right where you want to be."

"Yeah, I guess you're right, Mom. Thanks for listening—*Gee over!*—Love you," I say as the dogs take the command to turn to the right.

Deciding to stick with the program, I stop long enough to snack the dogs with sheefish, change their booties, and go. Their pace is now steady at about eight and a half miles per hour as we make our way back to Tuluksak. We aren't fast, but we are moving. More important, we are a team that doesn't quit. At long last, the Bethel finish line comes into view. I breathe a sigh of relief and feel huge pride for the dogs who see this race through to the finish.

At the K300 banquet on Monday evening, twenty-four hours after most mushers complete the race, I notice a few common themes. First, mushers agree that the trail conditions were the second worst ever witnessed, outranked only by the 2008 race now nicknamed the KuskoSwim. Second, most mushers confess to swearing to themselves that they will never race this course again. In the next breath, those same mushers also admit that, in hindsight, it wasn't all that bad. They will be here next year. The ability of mushers to have selective amnesia amazes me.

The challenge that the trail conditions posed made this race crazy, hard, and scary for a newbie like me. Rookie races demonstrate the importance of double and triple checking your actions, having great checklists, and wearing a bright headlamp. They teach new mushers about dealing with changing trail conditions, knowing the difference between a tired dog and a dog that is no longer having fun, and how our confidence level gets passed on to the dogs, for better and for worse. I laugh to think about the odd things that occur after being deprived of sleep and worn out. These lessons will be important as I prepare to run "the Last Great Race," the Iditarod.

▸LEAVING

ELY, MINNESOTA | 2000

Stilling the ripples.
Fish swimming at lake's bottom.
Lotus greets the fish.

—JOURNAL ENTRY, AUGUST 7, 1999

I call Dad. If I see him, I will cave and not be able to ask for help. I won't be able to leave.

"Dad, I need to buy a van. I am driving to Alaska. Can you help me find something? I have only a little money. There has to be something that can make it up there." I cross my fingers and hope he understands where I am coming from. I worry he will get protective or stubborn and say, "Heck no!"

"Dad, I need you right now. More than I ever have. I need to get my life on track. You and I both know Alaska is waiting for me. I have to get there somehow."

"Alaska? When do you need to go?"

Being on the phone, I am free to cry. Despite how much it hurts him to see me go, he will help. His quiet, nonjoking manner signals he is holding back his own feelings.

"Thank you, Dad. As soon as I can." I picture all the times we have spent over campfires, him dropping me off to ski on northern Minnesota winter trails, him walking me down the aisle on my wedding day. He always knows who I am.

"Dad, I don't want to go. I am lost without you, but I have to do this."

Dad finds an upgraded short bus for sale by a vendor who frequents the apartment complex where he works. Painted white, it has stickers along its sides with pictures of Pokémon ice cream bars. The horn still plays cartoon theme music that summons kids from miles away, hungry for frozen treats. Dad negotiates the price on my behalf. I pay $500.

A few days later, instead of ice cream, the bus now contains all my possessions—at least the ones important enough to bring with me. Some include Edward Abbey's novel about environmentalist sabotage, *The Monkey Wrench Gang*, and *Jonathan Livingston Seagull*, Richard Bach's fable about self-perfection. I have a stack of eighty-cent college-ruled notebooks I burn through as journals at a pace of one every three days. I bring my titanium ice ax from the Pacific Crest Trail, figuring it can offer me protection in a wide variety of situations. I shove all that, along with some clothes, food, a harmonica, and a mattress, into the back. There are curtains over all the windows, which makes it a comfortable, homey, and private abode—even if their multicolored, multipatterned vertical stripes make it look like a '60s living room frozen in time, complete with orange shag carpet. The bus averages eight miles per gallon, meaning I need more gas money for the full trip north, if it can make it at all. Dad looks over the engine and gives me a thumbs-up, which is the most I can hope for (see fig. 12).

Mom does not know of this plan. I drive the ice cream truck up north on a family trip, with Mom, her new husband John, Cindy, Cassie, and J.T. We stay at a cabin in Ely, a lakeside town in northeastern Minnesota. One evening I spring it on Mom that I won't be staying for the whole vacation—or coming home.

Mom tries to accept the reality of me leaving as we sit on the deck overlooking the lake, watching shapes form in the clouds drifting across a blue sky preparing for twilight. Highlighted by the setting sun, the western cluster of clouds fade from black to gray to gold to white. Within the Vermilion Iron Range, the deep-blue lake is surrounded by mineral-rich rock outcroppings. The burgundy rock reflection on the lake complements the wide range of red hues in a magnificent display of the setting sun. The terrain is thick with pines and cottonwood and is peppered with cottages where families watch the evening unfurl. I drink in every moment with Mom I can before setting out on my own. A large part of me is still this frightened girl clinging to her mom, daunted by the overwhelming unknown journey ahead of her.

After long, agonizing moments, Mom asks me, "Can you tell me again why you are leaving?"

I wish I had a better answer for her.

"Mom, I can't say why I am going. I am pulled along on a puppet string by a force much larger than I am." I select my next words with caution. "You taught me to be my own person. I know where my destiny resides, and every decision that takes me away from it pushes me further away from who I am. I am so disconnected right now, I don't even know who I am."

"Are you running away from something or running toward something?"

"I'm sorry. It must seem like I am running away. I only got out of treatment four months ago."

"That is putting it lightly, Katie. You were in a total dark period and hurting yourself. There are better ways to deal with life's challenges than leaving everyone you know behind."

"Mom, I know this is hard, but please trust me. I love you. I am going to Alaska, in part, to leave the darkness behind. More so, I am running toward a dream of who I want to be."

"You are my butterfly. Because I love you, I will set you free," she says.

As I tell J.T., he has worry across his face.

"Are you sure of this?" he asks.

I nod my head with more confidence than I feel. "I will not argue with whoever or whatever is guiding me to leave. After all we've been through, it is enough to look forward to tomorrow."

J.T. understands what I am saying. He has always been my confidant. I don't have to act strong in front of my brother. He knows me better than anyone. We enjoy long talks over green tea, deliberating about the meaning of life, quantum physics, programming, Buddhism, and just about anything. I will miss him.

"We don't always get the privilege to agree with what life throws in our path," he says.

I again nod in agreement. "Yeah, this dream of driving to Alaska has grown larger and larger each day until it encompasses my every thought." My gut clenches in knots as I say this, knowing the sadness I am causing my family by choosing to leave.

It is hardest saying goodbye to my little sisters. Cassie is only ten, and Cindy is eight. They need a hero for a big sister. Only a few months ago, I was sitting on a bus writing them a suicide letter. I am leaving and feel as though I have failed them. I hate myself for this.

I tell them, "Girls, I hope I can be a hero in your eyes again. I will live my life to the fullest and pave the way so I can show you how. Have the courage to follow your dreams."

Starting a new adventure, I lack any idea of where this path will lead. On July 16, 2000, I hit the road.

▸ALASKA OR BUST

KLUANE LAKE, YUKON TERRITORY | 2000

To find yourself. Think for yourself.

—SOCRATES

I am on a quest to Alaska to save my life. I want to be that ten-year-old girl again—the one who finds simple joy in the wilderness around her and loves exploring what is around the next bend.

Three days into my journey, the road ahead feels full of promise. With each passing mile-marker, I replace knots of apprehension with exhilaration and a courage born of confidence. My heart longs for crisp air, snow, rushing rivers, and tall pines. The open road leads to the horizon and to my future. No voices to hear and nothing to see but large fields of yellow canola flowers. Road trips have an inherent power to purge mental toxins. There is no way to avoid your mind. Nowhere to hide. The words of Jean Aspen echo in my daydreams and become clearer with every mile.

I overnight in Wal-Mart parking lots or pull into rest stations, where I can stay without trouble. On a whim, I pull off to the side of a dusty gravel road that makes up part of the Alaska Highway. I sit cradled in pure unadulterated silence for over thirty minutes before a loaded logging truck interrupts my requiem. The northwestern territories redefine wilderness, stillness, and grandeur. The valley ahead opens to the Canadian Rockies.

The setting sun gives a golden hue to snowcapped peaks. The eternal horizon features a story in which a golden knight duels with a crimson fire dragon, each struggling for control over the dawn sky. Blood-red balls of fire fly from the dragon's mouth only to deflect off the knight's impregnable gold shield.

My heartbeat quickens and laughter erupts from my belly. A loud, freeing laughter releasing years of stress and pressure. This is where I am meant to be. I scream with utter wild abandon at the top of my lungs then howl like a wolf toward a full moon on a cool night. The small worries and concerns fade away with the falling rain and the cleansing wind that cause the pines to dance before my eyes as one end of a full rainbow touches down twenty-five feet from me. Gazing out at the black-green pines, green grass plains, and deep-turquoise lakes, I am struck by the stillness. I have fallen into nowhere, at the center of everything. The wilderness has made its way back into my heart. Thank you, Dad, for planting the wild in my heart. Thank you, Mom, for nurturing it.

I settle back into the driver's seat of my Pokémon-speckled, '60s-living-room bus and keep on driving. Five days after I leave Minnesota, I encounter Teslin Lake, seventy-five miles long with cool-gray snowcapped mountains rising from its shoreline. A mother bear shuffles her two newborn cubs across the narrow, mud-filled dirt road.

As the changing landscape rolls by outside, varying thoughts roll through my head, reflecting the true transitory nature of the mind's endless chatter. Why do I put so much stake in one thought or feeling when I know it will pass? Recalling Buddhism lectures, I consider how thoughts and emotions enter and then leave, rising and falling upon the prevailing winds with no rhyme or reason. If you base an entire life upon those winds, you will lose your way. I contemplate how sailors use temperamental winds to cross a body of water and how surfers learn to toy with the waves as they roll in and out. I need to learn how to ride the waves of my consciousness while it dips in and out of the pools of thoughts and feelings. Perhaps then I can prevent myself from drowning in the ocean of my emotions or getting lost in the windstorm of my mind. All is impermanence.

A deep healing takes place far away from doctors, therapists, and self-help books. It takes a willingness to let go of your pained past and other defining attachments. Allow yourself to be free and swept up into the womb of all that exists. This is where empowerment exists, and life begins.

As each mile takes me further away from the nightmares invading my life, I feel the relief of change, release from the many unhealthy habits that have been haunting me. The scenery rolling past my window spurs memories of all the places I've explored over the past six years. I always imagined myself an adventurer, and my compulsion to roam has taken me to remarkable spots, full of natural beauty and history.

I camp beside Kluane Lake, in southwestern Yukon. Its thirty degrees Fahrenheit, and the sun sets at one-thirty in the morning only to rise again two hours later. I have entered a hall of kings. Maybe I read *The Lord of the Rings* too many times as a kid, but the immense landscape in Kluane National Park feels like a true last frontier with unmapped areas to explore.

Snow covers the dull, creamy gray of the mountain slopes, which run into chopped-up light-silver glaciers ending in a glossy snow-covered moraine, reminding me of the hundred-some-odd words the Inuit people use to describe snow. The land is an endless wonder, providing inspiration. Every nook and cranny showcase Mother Earth's attention to detail, from the smallest piece of grass to the largest mountain. The wildlife is more bountiful than the human population.

Log cabins along the road offer a convenient and economical way to live. The tree line reaches one eighth of the mountain height. The mint-green water of Kluane Lake bespeaks complete purity. Magenta and white flowers speckle the shoreline's rock beach. I have not seen color equal to these lakes since the Mediterranean.

Three thousand miles later, I cross the Alaska border, my quest a success. My body, mind, and spirit are more connected and alive than anytime since the PCT. I want to live to see tomorrow. A big old grizzly bear crosses the road, sauntering to the other side as if nothing else exists. Perhaps he is correct.

▸WEALTH

MATANUSKA GLACIER, ALASKA | 2000

A prayer flag which reads "Om Mani Padme Hum"
Dances in the autumn wind.

Is it the flag that moves? Or is it the wind?

Neither... it is your mind.

—JOURNAL ENTRY, DECEMBER 20, 2000

The Al-Can Highway crosses the border to Tok. From Tok, the road splits northwest to Fairbanks or southwest to Anchorage. I head toward Anchorage knowing I am short on money for gas and food. I pull over at the quaint Sheep Mountain Roadhouse and visit with other travelers while deciding where to go next.

Sitting outside the roadhouse, I pick up a paper to look at the want ads and end up reading my horoscope. It tells me "Last week's trip tapped into both heaven and hell. They are two sides of the same coin. Is it all perception? Must you realize hell before appreciating heaven?" I laugh out loud and earn strange looks from tourists.

This trip has been quite an emotional roller coaster. One minute my soul is flying higher than the distant peak touching the stars; the next, I am lower than the deepest crevasse, begging for mercy. The only consistency lies within change and turmoil. Grief holds tragic beauty.

moments of sadness are healthy for the soul, reminding us to be ... Freedom and authenticity courses through my heart.

I overhear a few nearby travelers conversing about wealth.

A guy with dreads says, "This land brings me to question society's definition of wealth."

"What do you mean? a girl with a long hippie skirt asks, "Wealth is wealth, and we sure don't have it!"

The group laughs.

He persists: "Think about it. The suburbs of Chicago or Beverly Hills, where money is everywhere, is in stark contrast to this land of so-called poverty. How do people even earn a living here? There isn't much financial opportunity."

A third man jumps in. "That's true. In fact, the money earned per square inch is too infinitesimal to account for."

"Yes! But here is my point," Mr. Dreads says. "This land has far more wealth than Beverly Hills can imagine! Wealth is in these gorgeous mountains, the trees, freedom, fresh air, and contentment. In Beverly Hills, this wealth is rare. In Alaska, it is all they know." His point made, he sits back down on the curb to bask in the sun's warmth.

Intrigued, I walk over and ask Mr. Dreads, "Do you think it's possible to keep this feeling of freedom with you even if you live in a city?"

The girl replies, "No way, dude! That's why we have to move here!"

Everyone laughs and nods in agreement.

I try again. "What about with meditation? Can't you find that freedom and wealth by searching for deep inner silence and connection? So that whether you are in Beverly Hills or on a glacier, you have that same freedom and wealth?" I didn't know the answer but was hoping one of them might.

I try to do Buddha justice. "During meditation, you connect to what is going on inside. It gives you a deep inner silence. You can tap into the core of all that's floating around in your consciousness. Catch it, pin it down, and let it go. We can have true freedom if we break the cycle of suffering and delusion."

The group looks puzzled at my explanation.

"How does that give you wealth?" Dreads asks.

I raise my shoulders. "I don't know!"

We all laugh and enjoy the freedom that comes with having no place to be and no agenda.

"Have you heard about the Wheel of Life?" I say.

The group jester says, "Wheel of Fortune? That's my Grandma's favorite show!"

Undistracted, my brain still tracks this line of thought. "If we get off the Wheel of Life that is where we find wealth."

Mr. Dreads tilts his chin. "What is on the Wheel? How do you get off?"

"Well, on the outside of the Wheel is the twelve-link chain of causation," I say. Inside the Wheel are six realms: heaven, jealousy, animal, hell, hungry ghosts, and human. I guess we spend time in these realms, fading in and out of them based on our mental state. You get off the wheel by not playing the Wheel of Life—like not clinging to our idea of self as if we are a fact."

"Huh, sounds promising," he says.

The girl jumps up. "Hey, come on a Matanuska Glacier tour with us! Our friend is taking us out, so it's free!"

"Yes, score!" I jump up at my great fortune. Counting my remaining dollars, I hope for enough to enjoy ice cream while we wait. Wealth and I don't coexist. No ice cream for me if I plan on being in Anchorage.

Glaciers are so foreign. You walk on crampons as if in moon boots. Looking deep into crevasses and holes leading into the center of the earth with water rushing through them to the underworld land of no return. I want more. I intend to use my time here well, however long that may be. The snow and ice are exhilarating. Adrenaline rushes to my head as I toe-pick over a large waterfall and steep slope. How much fun it would be to play forever in these cracks and holes of the crevasses. Sun glares off the surface of the ice. Ten thousand years ago, the glacier crept its way up the Mat-Su Valley. Two hundred and fifty thousand years ago, the glacier was in Anchorage. Such a length of time is incomprehensible.

▸SEA

SEWARD, ALASKA | 2000

Never lose an opportunity of seeing anything beautiful.
Beauty is God's handwriting.

—CHARLES KINGSLEY

I am at the end of the road in Seward, Alaska and out of money. I can only drive my ice cream truck about five miles more before it is out of even fumes. It is hard to worry about much. I am in the most beautiful place on the entire planet, nestled on the shores of Resurrection Bay, with massive mountains sliding into the glacial-blue water. The sky is vast and clear. Snowcapped mountains surround the sea. The setting sun casts an alpine glow on glaciers across the bay, painting them in orange.

The town itself is in the corner of the bay where historic Seward, established in 1904, showcases a long history of geology and mining. Hundreds of sea gulls circle around the sailboats and fishing vessels, exploring the sky realm uninhibited. A large whale welcomes me with its black-and-white fin splashing in the bay. Seward sits in a temperate rain forest, and vegetation abounds.

Mountains can make you feel either very lonely or very connected. Each range has a unique vibe to it. Here they are soft and welcoming, opening the heart of this ancient land to my foreign soul. Nature offers lessons for those who will listen. My ears experience a harmonic ecstasy with wave after wave breaking upon a rocky shoreline. Soft, mischievous winds toy with my hair, making me smile.

My soul can take a break from pushing along my path. This is it. I will stay here for the summer. I land a job at the Icicle Seafoods processing plant, starting out as a belly-slitter. Excited to have a job, I forget to consider what the job actually entails. The stench is overwhelming, and the wet work is tedious. I don't know what to expect on the "slime line." Perhaps my years of being a vegan have not prepared me for the harsh reality of Alaskan work. I walk away, after one day, with an eight-hour paycheck. I cash it and treat myself to a trip to the grocery store and gas station.

I continue my job search and discover a couple of kayak businesses in town that cater to local tourists. I stop in at one to find it staffed for the summer. They point me toward Alaska Kayak Company out on Lowell Point two miles south of Seward. Saving gas, I walk there to meet with an elderly gentleman named Jack.

"So, do you know how to kayak?" he asks.

"Sure! Yes, of course."

"Where did you learn? Do you have much sea kayaking experience?"

"I grew up in the Land of Ten Thousand Lakes. I lived on the water," I say, not answering his question. I've never been sea kayaking before. I canoed all over Minnesota, though—how different can it be? "I need work. I'm a super hard worker and love being on the water ... I'll do chores around the office. Please, give me this dream job."

"Let's get after it then," Jack says.

Puzzled, I follow him down to the beach.

"Let me see you suit up."

My blank stare as he hands me a kayak squirt, paddle, and life jacket answers a thousand questions.

"Hop in," he says. "I'll push you off."

Being on the water in this fast, slim sea kayak is exhilarating. We take off for a two-hour trip from the Lowell Point State Recreation Area to Tonsina Point. It must be obvious that I am not an expert kayak instructor. Jack gives me pointers on how to paddle. In my mind, the worst-case scenario is that I get a free kayak ride in Resurrection Bay—a win-win opportunity. It turns out that Jack has a soft spot for adventurers and gives me a job.

"I should let you know, while I am not homeless, I live in an ice cream short bus," I say. "Do you have a place I can park it?"

Jack nods in understanding. "You can park it alongside the office. There's a freezer in back, so help yourself to the food. Hope you like meat."

After starving for the past couple of weeks, this is a major gift. Tears of gratitude fill my eyes. I open the freezer to find it filled with frozen game: moose, halibut, and salmon. My days as a vegan are over.

I run over and give Jack a bear hug. "Thank you so much. I won't let you down."

Life can't get much better. I am on the water all day. The kayaking around Resurrection Bay features turquoise-blue waters, cracking glaciers, cliffs with nesting birds, puffins, bald eagles, leaping salmon, sea otters, harbor seals, killer whales—everything. I love taking tourists to isolated beaches and making a fire out of driftwood. Plus I get tips for doing what I love. Jack allows full access to the kayaks. At night, after everybody goes home for the day, I kayak around Resurrection Bay and explore in solitude.

▶ PHOSPHORESCENCE

SEWARD, ALASKA | 2000

There's a part of me, wild and free.
In my heart there's a wild wolf howling
through the tall pine trees.

It's a long cold trail that I've been on,

There just doesn't seem to be an end to this
way I've been going.

—HOBO JIM, "WILD AND FREE"

I am twenty-two years old today.

To celebrate, Jack tells me, "Why don't you take a kayak downtown. Young gal like yourself must enjoy a good time."

"I'd love to, Jack, but we have an early group tomorrow. I don't think I want to have a hangover on the choppy sea."

"Ah, the good old days," he says. "Don't you worry about that. I have it all planned out. Another guide offered to grab the morning trip for you."

I take him up on it, and as the sun sets, I push the single kayak into the still waters of the black ocean and paddle two miles to downtown Seward, where I pull the kayak high up on the shore, knowing the tide is coming up. I walk through downtown and let my ears follow the music. It is about ten at night and the action is just kicking in at the local joints.

I look for a place that matches my dancing style. I wander into the Yukon Bar, which seems to be a popular place. I grumble about the five-dollar cover but hand it over.

When he takes my ID and sees it is my birthday, the checker says, "Happy Birthday! Your drinks are on the house tonight!" In Alaska, women are few and far between, so we get treated accordingly. There is a saying about Alaska and its men: Where the odds are good, but the goods are odd. But I am not there to drink or look for men. I want to dance.

Dancing to good music brings a feeling of freedom. A man by the name of Hobo Jim is playing Alaskan music. His words generate pride in belonging in this great state, although my resident status is still pending. He plays songs about the Iditarod, living in wood cabins, being wild and free, the land of the midnight sun, the northern lights, and everything I am looking for in life. I stay all night. The "Iditarod Trail Song" appears to be a town favorite, and he plays it a handful of times.

The drunken crowd yells out in unison at every chorus, "I did, I did, I did the Iditarod Trail!"

I think to myself that one day I will sing this with conviction. My dream of being behind a team of dogs comes alive again. Thanks, Hobo Jim.

At one in the morning, I walk back to where I pulled up the kayak, and pause in wonder at the surrounding splendor. "Wild and free" is what I feel. I sit in the kayak, with the cold water of Resurrection Bay dripping onto my legs and push off the shore into glass-calm water. I take my time, wanting to linger in the solitude of the vast ocean water. I paddle through the thick liquid, reluctant to disturb the ocean's slumber. Making my way deeper into the bay, I stop paddling to lie back and stare up at the bright, starry sky sparkling with life.

The paddle dips into the water, which comes alive with color. This neon–blue-green magic substance shimmers every time I touch it as if fireflies are swimming in the water. Perplexed, I look behind me and see the kayak is leaving a trail of blue light. What did I drink tonight? This bioluminescent plankton is cheering me on or warning me away. The stars reflect in the water and a meteor shower adds to the glory like a cymbal punctuating a symphony.

A family of sea otters swims in front of the red kayak on their way to the shore. I watch them cross before daring to move again. My meditation stops when a larger-than-life whale rises in front of me and dives back into the water with a tail that flaps down into the water, splashing me with star-speckled water. The magic plankton soon scatters and the light dissipates, leaving me again in dark wonder.

It is my birthday, so I take all these experiences as a gift from the universe. I feel out of time and reality as I paddle back to my short bus of a home and sleep away my fairy-tale evening with visions of whales, dog teams, lead dogs, and 1,049 miles of the Iditarod Trail.

Part Two

ROOKIE MISTAKES

▶IDITAROD, MILE 0
ANCHORAGE, ALASKA | 2014

Away up in Alaska
The state that stands alone
There's a dog race run from Anchorage into Nome
And it's a grueling race with a lightning pace
Where chilly winds do wail.
Beneath the northern lights, across snow and ice
It's called the Iditarod Trail.

—HOBO JIM, "THE IDITAROD TRAIL SONG"

The Iditarod began during the famed diphtheria-serum run of 1925 when Leonhard Seppala and other dog mushers carried medicine across Interior Alaska to Nome in western Alaska. To commemorate the serum run, they held the first official Iditarod Trail Sled Dog Race in 1973. Mushers traveled, and still travel, from checkpoint to checkpoint much as freight mushers did ninety years ago. Joe Redington Sr., the Father of the Iditarod, organized the first Iditarod. His vision was to preserve sled dog culture, Alaskan huskies, and the historic Iditarod Trail between Seward and Nome. Joe and countless others made this cause their life's work. Out of respect, Joe's name is still called out during the roll call of every Iditarod Trail Committee board meeting. The board president excuses Redington's absence because "Joe is on the trail."

The Iditarod covers the roughest, most beautiful terrain Alaska offers. The official race starts in Willow. Mushers head out to the Yentna Station Roadhouse, Skwentna and then up through Finger Lake, Rainy Pass, over the jagged Alaska Range and down the other side to the Kuskokwim River. It leads into the interior and on to the mighty Yukon River, a highway that leads teams west. The trail goes through frozen rivers, tundra, and forest.

The race route alternates every other year. On even-numbered years, the trail heads north through Cripple, Ruby, and Galena. On odd years, the trail heads south through Iditarod, Shageluk, and Anvik. Teams end up following the Bering Sea coast through Unalakleet, Shaktoolik, Koyuk, Elim, Golovin, White Mountain, until at last arriving under the Burled Arch of Nome.

According to Bruce Lee from the *Iditarod Insider*, "Team building, that's what the Iditarod is all about." The race is unique in that there are thousands of trail volunteers, fifty-five volunteer veterinarians, and fifteen veterinary technicians.

As I gear up to run my first Iditarod in 2014, I focus not on competing but on learning how to run a long-distance race. My dog team has a wide age range with varied experience. Four dogs are between six and nine years old: Summit, Rambo, Huffy, and Speckle. Seven other dogs from our kennel are between two and four years old: Ears, Neo, Joy, Ghoulie, Ringo, Blaze, and Spook. I keep fourteen dogs, rather than the allowed sixteen, considering the difficult trail conditions this year. The race officials predict a hard, icy, and fast trail. More dogs could be unmanageable for a rookie. Ears and Summit are my core lead dogs.

The Iditarod auctions off the main seat in each mushers' sled during the ceremonial start in Anchorage, which goes twelve miles on city trails to the Campbell Creek Science Center. The Iditarod calls these auction winners "Idita-riders." A dog handler rides the second sled for safety in case a musher falls off the main sled during the downtown portion of the event and creates a risk for both the dogs and the Idita-rider. We don't want to give anyone too interesting of an experience.

"Are you ready?" I holler to the handler, hoping to hide my nervousness as I look down the starting chute on Fourth Avenue at one of my life's dreams. I do my best to keep calm and on top of things.

"Holy Shit!" I say under my breath so no one around me hears. I raise my head to look up at the Iditarod start banner and hear hundreds of dogs barking around me in eager anticipation of the run ahead.

"And here we have Katherine Keith from Kotzebue, Alaska," the announcers call out. Our team moves forward to line up at the starting chute.

"We made it!" I call out to anyone who will hear, not shy about embarrassing myself. At least my exclamation missed the TV cameras surrounding us while the announcers read the short bio of our team.

"Katherine is an iron woman. She and her dogs train year-round above the Arctic Circle with John Baker to have the best kennel in the world!"

I grimace, wondering why I don't pay better attention to what cheesy stuff I write in the bio.

The restart begins in Willow the following day at two o'clock. This is a far more serious event because it is the last opportunity to pack critical gear and get everything right, but I am fortunate to have a great crew of family and friends to get me to the start line.

"Three, two, one, go!" the announcer shouts.

Volunteers release my sled to enable the dogs to sprint northwest to Nome. The first fifty miles of the race is a total celebration. Every half mile has a new bonfire with people who cheer us on and somehow call out our names. Fans hand out cans of beer, Rockstar drinks, hot dogs, and cookies (see fig. 13).

The first few checkpoints are full of teams, but there are still a surprising number of teams camped outside the checkpoints. My strategy for the first few days of the race is to keep the dogs on an even run-rest schedule. This means I run the dogs five hours then rest for five hours. If the run goes long, the rest needs to increase by same amount. The trail to Finger Lake is flat and smooth, at which point the trail climbs up into the Alaska Range to the Rainy Pass checkpoint.

My naïvety leaves me ignorant of what makes up a good trail. I accept each successive mile with nonjudgmental openness. I enjoy almost every mile of trail and every checkpoint. I cherish this awe-inspiring adventure of crossing Alaska with only myself, a sled, and the finest of dogs.

▶GLACIER

SEWARD, ALASKA | 2000

Keep close to Nature's heart...and break clear away, once
in a while, and climb a mountain or spend a week in the
woods. Wash your spirit clean.

—JOHN MUIR

The summer tourist season dies down in Seward, and I need to find additional work. Not long after listening to Hobo Jim, I come across another dream job at Godwin Glacier Dog Sled Tours, which gives sled rides on top of a nearby glacier. As part of the job interview, I take a helicopter ride up to the glacier with some tourists. The pilot has a horrible sense of entertaining himself at the expense of the stomachs of his passengers. At least he provides information about the glacier and the wildlife inhabiting it. We land on a surreal moonlike setting, and a tour guide provides guests with information about dogs and dogsledding in Alaska and prepares them all for rides. This tour guide, Dario Daniels, has finished the Iditarod and is raising money to do so again this year. The tourists and I receive a thirty-minute dogsled ride across the gorgeous glacier. It comes at the steep price of $500 per adult, but it is clear from the guests, with smiling faces full of exhilaration, that they feel this is a once-in-a-lifetime experience. Another win-win situation for me whether or not I get the job.

I meet the crew and get a tour of the facilities. I stay up on the glacier all day, going down with the last tour. By the end of the week, I receive notification that I am hired. I give Jack my notice and my heartfelt thanks. He has another guide who can pick up any remaining tours.

I learn how to feed the dogs and harness them and figure out their names. As any dog handler knows, the quickest way to learn is just by doing. I get thrown into the mix with directions to just keep busy. Days later, I am on the runners learning the commands for making a dog team move forward (*up up*), turn right (*gee*), turn left (*haw*), and to stop (*whoa*). I am like a little kid at Christmas because, once again, I land a job I can't believe I get paid to do. I love this crazy state.

The glacier-mushing job is soon ending, and I need work for the winter. The most practical place for this is Anchorage, where there are many job opportunities and places to park my ice cream bus. But being stuck in the city isn't the right choice for me. I came up north to find the real Alaska. Time for the Brooks Range and bush Alaska.

One of my favorite places for refreshments in Seward is the iconic Resurrect Art Coffee House. I stop in when I'm off the glacier for a good cup of coffee and culture. They have job postings and notifications of interesting things going on around town. The old church architecture combined with local artwork makes a stunning backdrop for the mix of Alaskans and tourists who find their way here. I order my trademark "homeless iced latte" and browse the ads as I wait for my coffee. I look up and notice one with potential:

HELP WANTED IN KOTZEBUE, ALASKA

Learn about running dogs above the Arctic Circle in rural Alaska. We provide room and board. Contact Ruth Iten for information.

That is all the information I need. I give Ruth a call and talk to her about what the job entails. They buy an airplane ticket and arrange transportation from Kotzebue to their camp. I sell my bus for a profit in Girdwood and make my way up to Anchorage, where I catch a flight to Kotzebue in late September.

►HORSES

FISH CREEK, ALASKA | 2000

Argue for your limitations,
and sure enough, they're yours.

—RICHARD BACH

Getting to the Itens' camp entails a one-and-a-half-hour flight from Anchorage to the coastal city of Kotzebue. Iñupiat people have called "Kikiktagruk" home for at least six hundred years, and it was the hub of ancient arctic trading routes long before European contact. The population of Kotzebue is close to three thousand people, 96 percent of whom are Alaska Natives. The community still has deep roots in subsistence hunting and fishing, an integral part of its seasonal activities. Its location is ideal, situated between the Arctic Ocean via Kotzebue Sound, Noatak River, and Kobuk River. Hotham Inlet, also known as Kobuk Lake, fills up the space between Kotzebue on the Baldwin Peninsula, the rivers, and Selawik Lake. Friends of the Itens pick me up and put me in a boat. We cross Kobuk Lake heading east on a metal skiff for two hours, which puts me twenty-five miles east of town at Fish Creek.

From the shores of Kobuk Lake, we trek across the tundra permafrost for three miles with black spruce surrounding open tundra that stretches to the distant mountains. I arrive at camp, nestled in a wooden oasis, surrounded by a meandering creek. The place is far more beautiful than

I imagined. The Itens have at least ninety dogs, thirty-five of which are puppies under six months old. Twenty-seven dogs are Iditarod competitors.

I arrive to find caribou skulls, fish heads, and a bearskin on the porch. A caribou, gutted, hangs outside the front door. It's like walking onto the set of an episode of *Grizzly Adams*, my all-time favorite TV show growing up. An ongoing challenge of my childhood was that the show aired at the same time as Sunday school. I'd petition my mom to stay home and watch, insisting that *Grizzly Adams* was teaching me far more about God than school ever could. Now, thirty miles from the nearest Catholic church, my lessons will go on uninterrupted. Freeze-up starts in two weeks. It will be a month for the ice to be thick enough to travel on. During that time, we cannot receive supplies.

Iditarod musher Ed Iten and his wife, Ruth, put me to work. They have two children, Quinn and Katie, eight and eleven years old. After spending a day sorting through hundreds of dog booties, I realize the mundane, mindless tasks and chores are all part of an intricate system vital to the main goal of dog racing. When I have my dog yard, I must know all this.

In off-hours, I have the chance to explore the vast land. Peter, a construction worker from Scandinavia, and I take two Icelandic horses on a four-hour jaunt through the tundra. We cruise up a nearby ridgeline to the west, follow it north until we cross Fish Creek, then continue northeast to a valley. My mount, Tova, is very headstrong but adjusts to riding well. Traveling across tundra tussocks is difficult. It is marshy and mucky, with islands of dry land few and far between. We lunch on smoked fish and cheese. Conversation with Peter is difficult due to his thick accent, making only the most superficial chats possible.

On the way home, I spot a couple of caribou, which turn into a herd. We tie up our horses and sneak down to the meadow. Peter pulls out his rifle and takes a successful shot. I watch as life escapes its body. Peter guts the caribou, then places its still-warm heart and liver in my hands to carry home. Since moving to Alaska, I abandoned my vegan ways for more affordable and practical eating. This animal will feed us for two weeks at least, which poses an ethical dilemma. Is subsisting on local game more ethical than buying a burger in the store? If I am taking the life of an animal to support my own, shouldn't I at least show it the respect of being a part of the process? Buddhism is clear on the matter: it is not acceptable to kill animals for food. But I also need to balance out moral precepts with my survival. My only recourse is to consider that when my life circumstances change, I will give back and make different choices, try to reset my Karmic debt.

Coming home, I finish chores. I scoop dog poop from the yard for two hours and socialize with the puppies. I run three groups of puppies: one onto the tundra via the dog trail, one to the ridge, and the tiniest pups out to the pond. After feeding ninety dogs, I presoak breakfast, then chop and stack firewood.

I hear the dinner call at nine thirty—early tonight. Caribou stew with biscuits nourishes my body. It is my night for dishes, and before me lies a monumental stack. Water is boiling on the woodstove. I pour it into two stainless-steel bowls: one to wash and one to rinse. I drag my sore body up to bed at eleven thirty, tired to the bone. Various aches and pains course through my body as I drift away to sleep. The next morning, my head pounds with exhaustion. Perhaps it is the quiet ringing threatening to replace everything I've known. My need to be alone, even here, surprises me. I look forward to the peace and solitude of winter running.

With camp four miles from the boat landing across tundra, there is no easy way to transport supplies until it snows. Gear gets carried on our backs, on horseback, or via dogsled. Today, horses will bring up the gear. It's a gorgeous fall day with a slight crusting of ice on the water puddles along the trail. I saddle Sodie and head to the beach. Coming back, wind blows the tarp securing the packages. Sodie spooks and throws off half the load before trying to run away. Lesson number one about getting horses to do the heavy lifting: tie stuff down.

Ed, Ruth, and I decide that building a round pen will establish a proper horse-training program to saddle-break the younger horses. A round pen requires two dozen fourteen-foot log poles. I start by digging postholes through a foot of frozen clay and permafrost. I haul up three buckets full of rocks and sand from Fish Creek, then cut down all the trees within the circle. The Itens have ten poles to get started with. We need a dozen more. The distance is too great to haul the remaining poles by woman power alone. Time for the horses to step up.

I begin the process by using Sodie to haul back the first pole. It is a hair-raising record trip. Sodie is unstoppable at a full sprint, hauling a tree behind and me on top. Upon arrival at the pen, I am shaking with adrenaline but happy to be back in one piece with a pole.

I take Sodie back for a second pole right away. We need to face our fears. Using a bungee, I tie the next log pole to her. She spooks, running in frantic circles around a tree. The pole flies off, and my already-swollen ankle gets kicked. We limp home without a pole, but the reward is a stunning orange moonrise.

Tova gets the next turn but doesn't want to cooperate. He feels higher up on the dominance chain so listens accordingly. Can't say he's wrong. This time, I hold on to the rope rather than tie it to Tova. Bad idea. Tova takes off, and the pole meets up with a stump. It catches, but Tova doesn't stop. The rope tightens around my hand, and my body flies off the saddle, leaving one of my big cold-weather waterproof boots still stuck in the stirrup. An unhappy ending.

Back in the saddle, I keep trying to hold the rope but it slips through my hands. I halt Tova to pick up a long stick to snag the stranded rope. This bad idea doesn't work and only results in me sprawling headfirst into a tree. Tova books it all the way back to the stables, leaving me alone to follow our trail during heavy snowfall. Not willing to give up, I elect to go on another painstaking pole ride. My punished wrist, sore and weak, cannot tighten the saddle as needed. I secure the log pole around the saddle horn this time. Halfway back, the saddle falls sideways, and off I go, straight into another tree.

I take the next two days teaching Tova to stop and stay with leg pressure commands. We now have five inches of beautiful powdery snow. At last, the magnificent freeze-up arrives. The mornings are darker, and the nights longer. I take Tova out and cut down a few more log poles with a chain saw. I rig up a hobble for him, and we walk all the way home without a pole to test it out. I fight a losing war with these huge horses. There must be a way to outsmart them, to beat them at their own game.

Ready for a pole, we try again. Tova and I fight for three hours in a sheer battle of wills. I get him near the log pole, and he slows down somewhat. The instant I touch the rope, however, he bolts, hell-bent for home. I yank with one arm on the hobble rope while the other arm tries to turn him around with the reins.

I tie Tova to a tree, so he can't move. I put the log on the saddleback, hop on, and get the hobble straight. For twenty minutes, I work to unhook Tova from the tree while I am on his back. The instant I do, wham! Off we go. My wrists are unable hold on, and we are out of control. We are halfway home in maybe five seconds. I lean far forward, my body weight off balance as I try to hold the hobble. Tova comes close to a tree, the branches come close to my face, and smack! Down I fall. I roll away to avoid the huge fourteen-foot pole Tova is dragging. I walk home, my head bowed, to find Tova waiting for me out at the pond with the other two horses. Happy to see he is not hurt, I backtrack to find the log that fell off about a mile away from the round pen. I bend down, put the spruce pole on my shoulders, and carry it to the pen myself. Way simpler.

I receive a mix tape in the mail from a friend who helped me during my hospital stay in Minneapolis. A year has passed since the cutting began, leaving still-visible scars. I remember lying in the hospital bed, listening to this soundtrack, hoping to find a place of peace where I might regain strength and sanity. Here, above the Arctic Circle, my life is no longer a living nightmare. The threat of self-extinction seems far off, obscure, and absurd. Certain words or phrases still trigger flashbacks, but they have become more manageable. Arctic solitude highlights all shortcomings and sensitivities. My thoughts can get trapped in the past, leading to a few days of total exhaustion, negativity, and pain. Dark periods exist, but instead of months they now last only days. I hope that perhaps even these will pass. Flashbacks and self-harm don't belong in the life I am building.

I study the art of running a team of dogs and surviving the Arctic winter. A month after I arrive, I drive a small dog team for the first time solo. Two weeks later I am on the runners of a fourteen-dog team. There is no turning back. The lifestyle completes me and transforms all my past goals and dreams into something better.

▸MUMMY

FISH CREEK, ALASKA | 2000

Could a greater miracle take place than for us to look
through each other's eyes for an instant?

—HENRY DAVID THOREAU

It's Halloween. Alexa, the neighbor girl, comes over, dropped off by her Tata Louie's dog team. A neighbor from ten miles away, David Keith, drops off his eight-year-old son, Alan, while I am busy with dog chores. Alan spends the day with us making Halloween preparations. Kobuk Lake is still freezing up, so no one can make it to town. This Halloween is without candy, so we plan a treasure hunt. I create clues and decorate them with colored paper. Ruth makes donuts and snow ice cream. We put out dehydrated apples and apricots.

I am out in the dog lot hiding clues as darkness descends. I hear a snow machine pull up away from camp. I am worried that someone is broke down or stuck. I hike out to investigate, when I spy a bulky mummy. I conceal my laughter as the tall, mysterious figure, wrapped with materials from a first aid kit, makes its way to the house. The mummy lingers outside the front door for over ten minutes until someone opens it. It roars in a deep baritone voice. Ruth screams! Chaos ensues as kids run out to see the mummy, laugh as they realize who it is, and unwind him to reveal a six-foot-tall gentle giant of a man.

I walk up to the cabin to get the treasure hunt started and introduce myself. The instant my eyes meet his, I fall in love with him—just like that. Staring into his eyes, I feel more at home than I have in my twenty-two years. Five seconds go by, then ten, then twenty.

I reach out my hand to introduce myself.

"Um … ah … hi. I'm Kat." I can't even talk.

He extends a long right arm to shake my hand. His warm, muscular hand grips mine in a firm shake that becomes something of an embrace. I imagine that same hand reaching out to grab my neck and pull me into a deep kiss full of longing and hunger.

"Hi. I'm Dave," he answers.

I continue to stare at his handsome, rugged face with a solid five o'clock shadow, maroon hooded sweatshirt, and KOTZ Radio baseball cap.

"Alan is a great kid," I say, cringing a little at my lack of originality. "I mean, he is so funny. His jokes are the best. He makes everyone around him happy."

My cheeks are hot as I blush. Still staring, I force myself to release his strong, safe hand. I don't want a day to pass without him. I want Dave to rescue me and save me from myself. He is the safe harbor that my rocky ship has been long searching for. I picture the rest of our moments together, the details upon which I will build my life. My future path lies parallel to his, poor guy. I wonder if he is ready.

Throughout the Halloween evening, there is so much laughter my sides hurt. Kate, Quinn, Alexa, and Alan all try bobbing for apples with their hands tied behind their back. They end up soaking wet. As the night progresses, I become enamored of Dave's easy laugh. Time flies by, yet everything seems to pause. He is an open person with a deep nature and an astute mind. Dave was born and raised in central Washington and is knowledgeable about any subject from archaeology to geology to mechanics. Dave is a single parent to Alan. They live at a camp about nine miles from the Itens on the north shore of Kobuk Lake (see fig. 14).

After Halloween, Dave comes over every day. I am enthralled during his visits, and afterward wait, without patience, for the next one. They come over for Thanksgiving. I take the entire day to cook, making everything from scratch. Dave arrives at two o'clock all cleaned up, better than the rest of us, with jeans and a T-shirt. My stomach flutters when I think of him and when we are close. When we talk, our eyes lock, and I get lost in the depths of silent communication. The solitude of camp life accentuates the feelings of a budding romance. I know something binds us. Doing what is as necessary as breathing, we have no choice but to fall in love.

▶IDITAROD, MILE 153

RAINY PASS, ALASKA | 2014

Well, give me a team and a good lead dog
and a sled that's built so fine,
And let me race those miles to Nome,
one thousand forty-nine
Then when I get back to my home
Hey I can tell my tale
I did, I did I did the Iditarod Trail.

—HOBO JIM, "THE IDITAROD TRAIL SONG"

The infamous Steps involve steep and technically challenging switchbacks. The Iditarod trail crew works hard to make the trail safe. Our team has no problems with the Steps, but others do. One musher, Jake Berkowitz, breaks his gang line, and the front fourteen dogs go down the Steps by themselves, followed by Jake with his sled pulled by two dogs. The *Iditarod Insider* catches this unfortunate situation on video to our great amusement.

It is clear upon arrival at the Rainy Pass checkpoint that the trail ahead to Rohn is dangerous and technical. The first mushers get injured or damage their sleds or both. The checkpoint officials recommend teams proceed with caution or consider staying in Rainy Pass. I alter my race strategy by cutting the team's rest in hopes they won't be at top strength going down through the Dalzell Gorge. Given the extremely steep descent through the Gorge, a strong team will turn uncontrolled chaos into disaster. Leaving early might also allow me to navigate more trail during daylight. The trail leaving Rainy Pass climbs high into the mountain pass until it arrives at the gorge. The low-snow conditions require days of hard labor by the Iditarod trail crew to make conditions passable.

"Martin Buser is first into Rohn and has a broken sled," a cold-looking volunteer says with an Alabama accent. He is trying to do me a favor by keeping me up to date with the latest trail information. "Plus, Scott Janssen even broke a leg."

My body tenses up as I try to decide if I want to listen or turn away and stay ignorant. I look to the mountains with a crystal-blue sky darkening under the weight of a setting sun that crashes into a deep orange horizon. Deep down, I can't wait to hit the trail. I get to run dogs through the Alaska Range—Who gets to do that?—fear or no fear.

"We've got this," I say to myself rather than the volunteer.

Unable to sleep, I walk up through the line of sleeping dogs to check on their breathing. Summit, the regal leader, is playing around, trying to dig up some old food buried in the snow. He seems interested in the female leader in the team next to him. His slate-gray fur stands up on the back of his neck as the male from that team notices Summit's interest and takes considerable offense. I sit on the straw next to him.

"Come here, old boy," I say to Summit, showing him that my lap is open. I reach down to massage his ears. He leans into me with quiet satisfaction as his body relaxes into the bed of straw.

"Attaboy," I say to soothe both his nerves and mine. If we can keep calm, happy, and confident, we will be much better off in the miles ahead.

I put booties on the dogs and get ready to go. Knowing we can't stop anywhere on the trail ahead, I carry a bag of meat snacks up to the front of the team and throw out a half-pound piece to each dog. They jump up, wag their tails, and bark. I check the condition of each dog and make sure their harnesses fit. I whistle to the team, asking them to stand up off the straw. Time to leave the checkpoint.

I call out "Gee!" and "Haw!" to steer the leaders to the trail heading toward the Alaska Range. Once on the trail, they know it. They put their weight into the harness, and enthusiasm ripples off them and rolls back into me. Regardless of what lies ahead, we will cope. The trail ahead holds nothing that can hurt me more than I have already. I dare this trail to beat me when life has yet failed to do so.

▸SHEEFISH

FISH CREEK, ALASKA | 2000

However many holy words you read,
however many you speak,
what good will they do you if you
do not act upon them?

—GAUTAMA BUDDHA

By the end of November, day three of forty-below temperatures, cold penetrates the house. Even inside, I wear two pairs of socks; three pairs of long underwear; four tops, including a fat sweater; and a hat. I am chilled to the bone. It is hard to stray from the woodstove. My nose is raw from overexposure. Dressing to go outside in this weather involves donning a massive, bulky suit, boots that are three times my usual size, a beaver-fur hat, a thick neck warmer, three glove liners, and huge travel mitts eight times my hand size that extend up to my elbow. I learn how to survive— no, thrive—in this harsh climate, this magical place. The atmosphere is exhilarating. Breathing alone provides a natural high.

We need fish. The dogs are getting skinny, and we use two bags of dog food daily. In the warmth of camp, over two days we weave floats and rope through the tops and bottoms of two 150-foot-long nets taking meticulous care to hang them in even intervals. Once finished, it is time to place them beneath the ice of Kobuk Lake.

Ed, his brother Mark, and Peter take two snow machines. Ruth, the kids, and I follow by dog team. Two hours later, we find them nine miles from camp on Kobuk Lake.

The giant, white sea leads out to the foreign horizon. The traditional process for placing sheefish gill nets under the ice is nuanced. We cut holes in the ice ten feet apart and thread a rope under the holes using a twelve-foot spruce pole with an antler secured to the tip as a hook. We do this for three hundred feet until the rope is all under the ice. Meanwhile, the temperature is ten below with harsh winds blowing in our faces. My gloves and clothes, now wet, quickly freeze solid, which makes holding on to an ice-covered tree pole a challenge.

After finishing the net, we run the dogs back to camp. The sun dips down below the icy horizon, and the full moon rises in the east in perfect counterbalance. A bright orange fireball sets the white ice on fire. The ice turns to molten lava as the moon creeps away from the edge of existence. Jupiter and Saturn shine, indifferent to our efforts and to the spectacular antics of the moon. The planets march their way through the zodiac, and one by one the stars add their light to the blackness of the heavens. This silent song sings to my soul. Frozen and numb, I enjoy the run home.

After feeding the dogs, I sit on the pond by the water hole again, looking up at Jupiter as it shines out, ascending in the north. Northern lights reach from west to east curving in a green arc. The outermost ring is a brilliant reddish orange. The lights follow the plane of the ecliptic. Perhaps, if I could stand on Saturn, this is what its rings would look like. I sit. Not a single thought floats through my consciousness. Sitting, taking God in, letting self go. Breathing. Breathing. Breathing. To maintain a healthy and strong mind, I have renewed my Buddhist practice.

My earlier Buddhist teachings follow me up north, but they now take a turn into *metta*, universal loving-kindness. In secret, I endeavor to be a great and humble bodhisattva, a spiritual warrior who delays reaching enlightenment so they can help others to get there first. This is who I want to be. I want to take my ugly trauma and transform it into a magnificent lotus flower from which all people can inhale the essence and heal in that instant. In this manner, my suffering may have meaning and may be worth it. No, I don't have an ego. But, yes, I want to ease suffering. Please let me help!

I want to be a torch, one that sparks inspiration and hope in others; a hermit in the night, wandering through the dark fog, lighting the way for lost and lonely travelers. I wish for others to say yes rather than giving up on themselves. All people should have someone in their life as I had Judith that night when, in a desperate state, I needed to hear that one strong word: live. That spontaneous answer was my truest gift. I am not a real believer in God. I try on religions like shirts in a thrift store. It isn't the shirt that matters but who wears the shirt. I've been an atheist, a shaman, a Buddhist, a Catholic, a new age spiritualist, a light worker, all within the first twenty years of my life. That *yes* changed me.

I understand that to be a bodhisattva, I need to gain *bodhicitta*, an awakened heart. An awakened heart is not a fake-happy thing. An awakened heart, while wounded, softens with an awareness of suffering. While out in the dog yard, feeding ninety hungry canines, I have time to recite the Four Noble Truths of Buddhism as if a mantra. "Suffering is a part of everyone's life. The cause of suffering is our own desire, ignorance, and hatred. We can extinguish desire by liberating ourselves from attachment. We can overcome suffering by following the Eightfold Path."

It is part of my master plan that living in the middle of the wilderness in "Nowhere, Alaska," will help me follow the Eightfold Path. It demands a commitment to be the best person I can be. In such capacity, maybe I can overcome suffering. It's that easy—eight steps:

1. Develop a deep understanding of the Four Noble Truths to inspire us to continue with the remaining steps.
2. Commit to self-improvement.
3. Speak in kind and truthful manner.

Okay, great. Steps one through three I have covered.

4. Develop "right action" through behaving with compassion toward others.

I wonder what this means. Does this mean compassion for my abuser? No thanks. I fall into the category of a nice Minnesotan. I will cook you goulash and tuna casserole and send you on your way. But yes, I *will* send you on your way. Plus, I might spit in your goulash.

5. Earning a living harming no being.

Where does dog mushing come in? I feed the dogs fish. It brings the fish harm to keep the dogs alive. Is that wrong? What about when the dogs injure their shoulders or wrists while racing? What about the horses? We ride horses, and they help with manual labor. Is that harming them? Also, since coming to Alaska, I've been eating a lot of meat. In fact, it is my main food group. I am going to hell. Oh, wait, this is not Catholicism.

6. Banishing negative thoughts to conquer ignorance and desires.

Wow, I am terrible at this. The Eightfold Path might be harder to follow than I think. I am the queen of hating myself. I hate myself so much that I was ready to kill myself. How does a person ever change being negative? I have been through tons of therapy and learned many skills, but my mental loop is the same as it ever has been.

7. Encourage wholesome thoughts. All we say and do arises from our thoughts.
8. Develop and strengthen the depth of our concentration.

Number eight seems to be the easiest.

I am a terrible bodhisattva and a terrible Buddhist to boot. Can we clean our slate? Can we erase karma? My mantra is now "May all beings be well; may all beings find happiness; may all beings be free from suffering; may I not be a loser." Humor helps.

I hear my stomach growl as I face the most difficult decision to date: Do I stay here outside, coexisting with hard-won, complete sanity, or do I go where dinner and wine wait? Realizing, the sky won't be going away, it doesn't take long before I am warming up indoors.

▸MOOSE

KOBUK LAKE, ALASKA | 2000

Stillness of the dead of night

Stillness between tides and waves

Stillness of the instant before creation.

—JOURNAL ENTRY, DECEMBER 9, 2000

At noon I take off to the sheefish net, nine miles away. My lead dog, Devon, has a different goal in mind. For two hours Devon insists on going the wrong way. Devon turns the team around at every opportunity. I tip my sled over twice and break two snow hooks. Realizing Devon is only interested in messing with me, I try other dogs up in lead, but none of them can lead the team. I have to turn around to get a different leader. Twenty minutes after getting back, Peter pulls up with the other good dogs. I grab two, putting Garrett in lead, and am relieved to find he is a perfect fit. We head out toward the net again with no problems. The temperature drops after I get to the nets. The brisk twenty degrees below zero now turns to minus thirty.

I want to visit to Dave's camp to say hi, use his jigsaws, and go sledding with Alan. Dave is leaving for three weeks for the Christmas holiday. It will be a long three weeks, but perhaps it will clear my head and let the butterflies in my stomach rest. After checking the net, I take the dogs another two miles to find an empty house and a locked door. I see my reflection in his window. I'm frozen. Ice covers my eyebrows and lashes. My hair is solid white. I get home, not once being inside for the past seven hours at thirty below. It takes over an hour for my face to thaw.

A week later I take my skate skis and start the ten-mile trek to Dave's camp. After calling ahead, I know he is home. I spot four new sets of moose tracks. Near the beach, I hear a moose call out in front of me. It sounds like a snow machine stuck in the snow, revving its engine to break out of its hole. I assume that it is a mom separated from her calf with me in between. Instead of bolstering my courage, my past close encounters with a mountain lion and bear only help me realize that I don't care to be in this situation again. I can't keep turning around only to feel stranded and alone, afraid to venture out anywhere. I need to learn to shoot a gun. I need to get to Dave's camp regardless, so onward. The three of us have a great time and say our goodbyes for the holidays.

Weeks pass by at a crawl. Dave's long absence from Kotzebue makes me eager to see him again. I spend New Year's Eve in Kotzebue to watch the fireworks as a treat. On the way back to camp, I stop at Dave's, aware he is home. It is a pitch-black night, cloudy with no moon. I make it to Dave's around eight o'clock in the evening. Alan is in town for the night. It is awkward at first, without Alan there to connect with or distract me, but Dave brings out the Wild Turkey, and any tension soon dissipates.

The music is blaring while Dave and I blabber on about everything and nothing. Throughout the night, we loosen up and let go of any blocks holding us back from getting close. Through our stories, I discover that Dave doesn't want marriage, because of how it binds and ties you down, how it restricts and suffocates. Dave discovers how I feel a relationship should be as two wholes coming together in freedom. In our own ways, we check out each other's perspectives.

By three in the morning, we figure out I am not leaving, and he offers me his bed. We lie next to each other's naked skin. Nothing feels finer, so comforting, so warm. It doesn't take long for our bodies to unite in passionate, mad lovemaking. We cling to each other in desperate craving for the union we've been longing for. Hungry for every inch of him, I won't let him go.

In the morning, Dave mentions his plans for the log cabin he is constructing, plans that now include me. I feel we will either slide into this courting-type situation, or I will move over to Dave's camp, starting a new life at once. Knowing myself, it seems likely I will be extreme.

After seven months of living at the Itens, I absorb all I can from them, and it is time to leave. Ed and Ruth provide me with a plane ticket to Anchorage. I pack my bags and get a ride via snow machine to Dave's camp. Dave isn't expecting me.

I pull up with my luggage and ask him, "Can I stay for a few days? Maybe a couple weeks while I decide where to find work?"

Dave says, "Want you to stay? Heck, I even have a chair with your name carved on it waiting for you. You are not going anywhere."

From that point forward, we wind up making our plans together (see fig. 15).

▸IDITAROD, MILE 188

ROHN, ALASKA | 2014

Well the race it won't be easy
For the masters of the trail
And some of them will make it and
some of them will fail
But just to run that race takes a
tough and hardy breed,
And a lot of work done by the dogs
that run across snow with whistling speed.

—HOBO JIM, "THE IDITAROD TRAIL SONG"

After a long, winding ascent to the 4,875-foot summit of Rainy Pass, we dip down into Dalzell Gorge. There is no snow. The trail is an endless vertical chute of dirt, glare ice, ice blocks, tree stumps, and rocks. Ice bridges exist, but half the time their angle swings me and the sled into a gully to smack into a wall of ice, stopping all progress. The danger is real. The sled brake and tracks need snow to be effective. I have little to no stopping power. The dogs know they have control, and it feeds their enthusiasm. Faster and faster we fly through the gorge. Every second of the trail requires full focus to balance on the sled and avoid tipping over and colliding headfirst with a tree. We crash our way down Dalzell Gorge, helpless to avoid catastrophe. Between moments of panic and adrenaline, I laugh with the pure joy that comes from being in a flow state, completely absorbed in this ultimate challenge. In the dark of night, the turns ahead are invisible. My hands grip the sled in expectation. Every ounce of strength and concentration is at my disposal. I don't know if the difficult part is over or whether another death-defying section is just around the bend.

I am ecstatic when I finally pull into the stately, pine-tree-surrounded Rohn checkpoint in one piece.

"How was the trail?" Bruce Lee asks upon my arrival.

"It was awesome!" I say, and I mean it too. I'm in a state of excited triumph and feel more alive than I have in years.

I feed and bed down the dogs, when exhaustion sweeps over me. I crawl into my sleeping bag next to the dogs on a pile of straw protected by a large pine. My body aches as I lay down to rest, feeling for the first time all the bumps and bruises from the run. At twenty below zero, I am warm enough. The smoke of firewood from tent frames combines with the fish from the dog cookers to produce a pure Alaskan aroma. I crawl deeper into my bag hoping for sleep. There are likely two hundred dogs in Rohn—all of them wired after the Gorge. Rounds of long, soulful howls roll across the checkpoint in waves as they join in a chorus of harmony.

After forty-five minutes of trying to sleep, I give up. I require coffee. I stumble into the checkpoint station to fill up my thermos.

I overhear Jake Berkowitz say, "The next run will be tough. It's just as challenging as the run we completed getting here."

My schedule calls for a four-hour rest, and I pace around the dog yard trying to keep from leaving early. Reports highlight over a dozen scratches from the race so far. In addition, the trail injures übertough mushers, some of whom are still racing. Hans Gatt flew into a tree and didn't know where he was. Ralph Johannessen broke ribs. Aaron Burmeister tore the ACL in both his knees. I see printed-out reports of people scratching. I'm uneasy, but I must continue.

The trail through the Farewell Burn has no snow either. I make it through the first five miles at a slow crawl. The uphill climbs have coarse sand that drags on the plastic sled runners. I push my sled up the hill, running alongside it. The sled gets caught on roots, rocks, and anything else that feels like it. The downhills on the frozen rock become steep, fast, long, and full of obstacles. The burn is worse than the gorge. I dance on the runners as my sled flies down one steep hill after another with no steering.

This continues until we bounce off one tree, hit a rock, then fly headfirst into another tree. Crack! Did my head hit the tree? Did my sled hit it? Dazed, I walk up to check on the team hoping they are okay. I walk back to the sled to resume our traveling.

"Up, Up," I call out.

Nothing happens.

"All right. Good dogs! Let's go! Up!"

Again, nothing happens. Maybe I hit my head harder than I thought.

▶LIVING

KOBUK LAKE, ALASKA | 2001

In the caribou tundra, in the wild barren land.
On the fierce arctic ice, where the polar bears stand.
Where the trail of the Eskimo hunter is worn.
This is the country where legends are born.
Where the northern lights blaze above a cold arctic
haze and caribou come to an old shaman's drum.

—HOBO JIM, "WHERE LEGENDS ARE BORN"

The serenity I find with Dave in the heart of this landscape I'd envisioned since I was a child feels too good to be true. Dave and I struggle to trust one another enough to become vulnerable. He comes to our relationship with his own baggage too, having been in a relationship with a woman who left him with sole custody of their now-eight-year-old son.

Alan has trouble adjusting to my presence in his life. I want to be his friend yet also a mother and teacher. Dave and Alan aren't keeping up with Alan's homeschooling. I encourage rebellious Alan to get his work done and take his required tests. Alan misses the solo time with his dad, but we find avenues to connect. We can play various games until the generator runs out of gas, the gas lights run out of propane, and Dave is snoring. Even then, we can stay entertained.

Chores take up a lot of time. Dave is an expert at working a chain

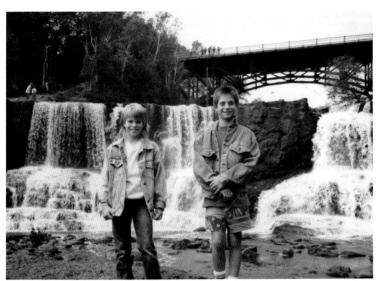

Figure 1
My brother,
J.T., and me at
Gooseberry Falls,
MN, camping
with Dad

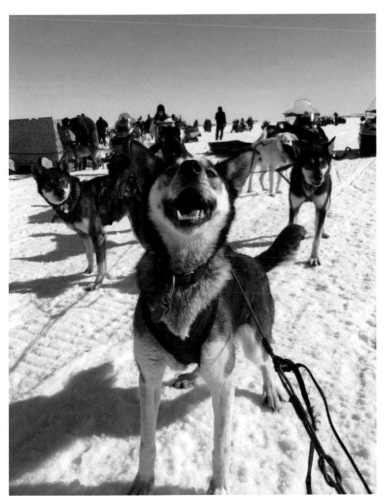

Figure 2
Ears prior to the
Junior Kobuk 440

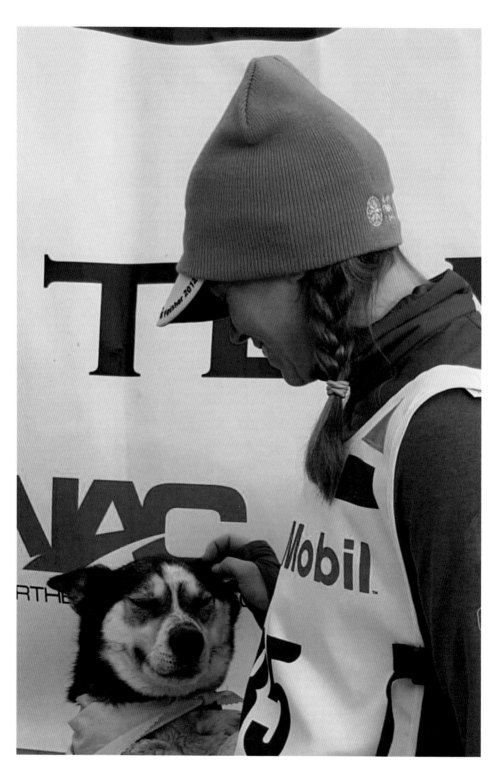

Figure 3
Ears showing some love prior to the Iditarod start

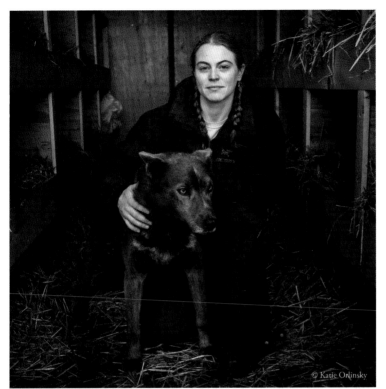

Figure 4
Summit posing for
the *New York Times*

© Katie Orlinsky

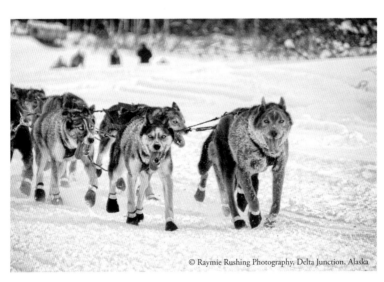

Figure 5
Ears and Summit
in lead

© Raymie Rushing Photography, Delta Junction, Alaska

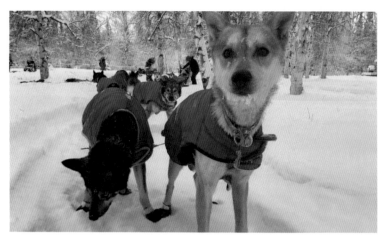

Figure 6
Blondie during the
Yukon Quest

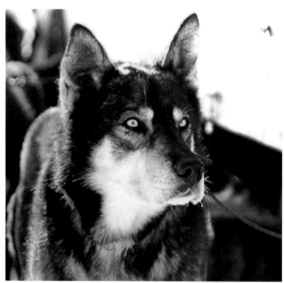

Figure 7
Rambo

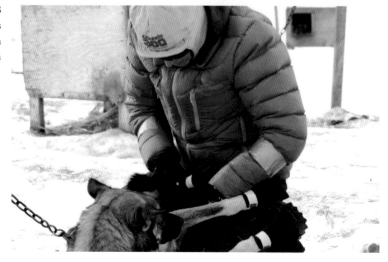

Figure 8
Putting booties
on prior to a
training run

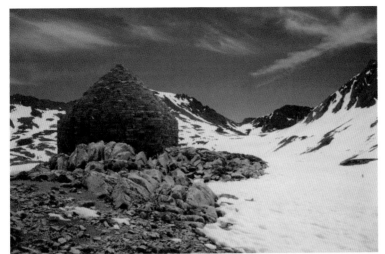

Figure 9
Muir Pass

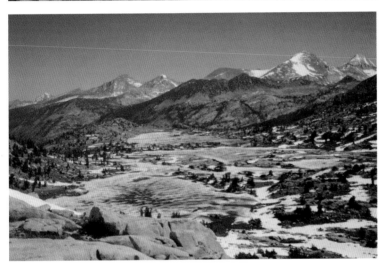

Figure 10
The climb down
from Sendall Pass

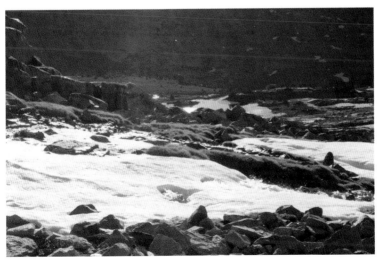

Figure 11
The trail to
Benson Lake

Figure 12
The short bus
ice cream truck

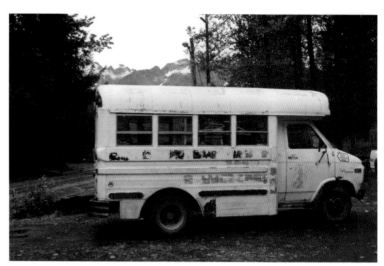

Figure 13
Leaving Willow
at the start of
Iditarod 2014

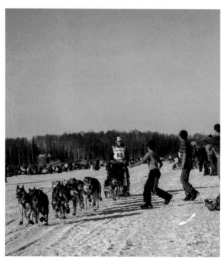

Figure 14
Dave and Penny
at camp

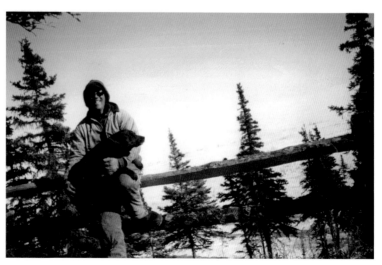

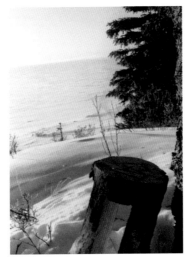

Figure 15
The stool made
by Dave as a
welcome gift

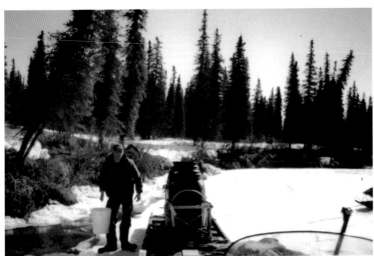

Figure 16
Hauling water
from the creek

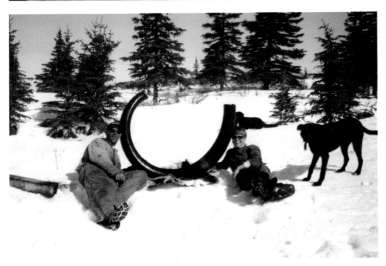

Figure 17
Mammoth tusk

Figure 18
Alan stacking
up sheefish

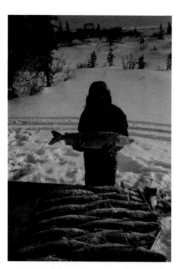

Figure 19
Framing the
log cabin

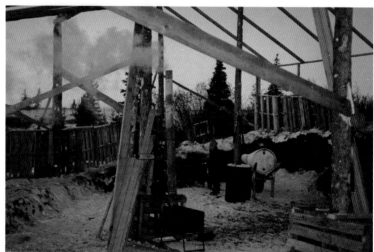

Figure 20
Pile of logs
behind the cabin

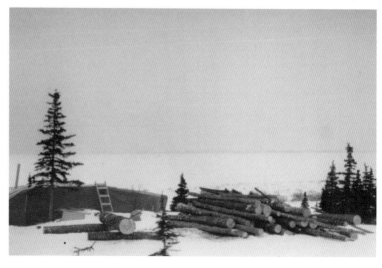

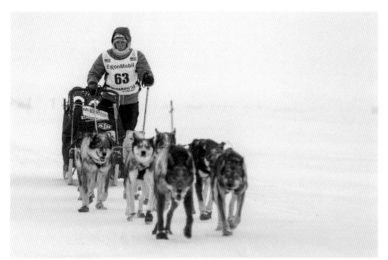

Figure 21
Coming up the sea
ice into Nome

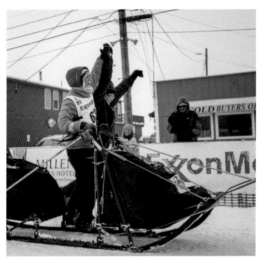

Figure 22
Crossing the finish
line with Amelia

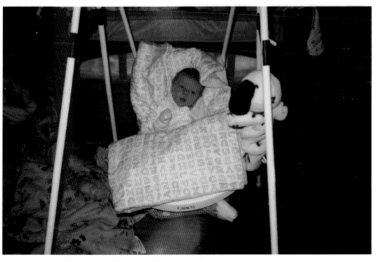

Figure 23
Madi in her swing
for the first time

Figure 24
At the ceremonial start of the 2015 Iditarod

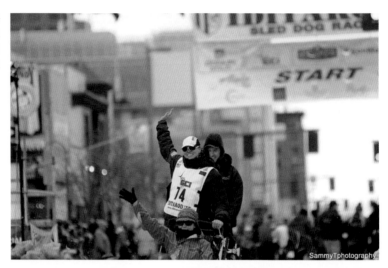

Figure 25
Dave and me standing by the casket we made for Madi

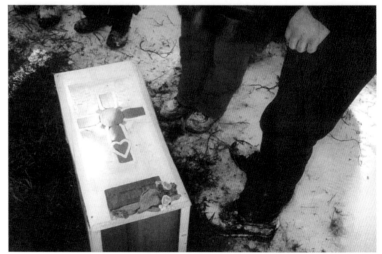

Figure 26
Wedding day

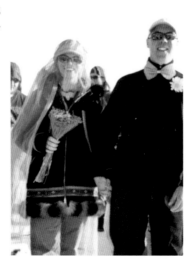

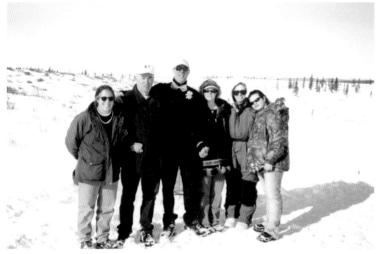

Figure 27
Left to right:
Angela Eisel (friend),
Dewey Keith
(father-in-law),
David Keith,
Kat Keith, Patricia
Byrne (mom), and
Cindy Foster (sister)

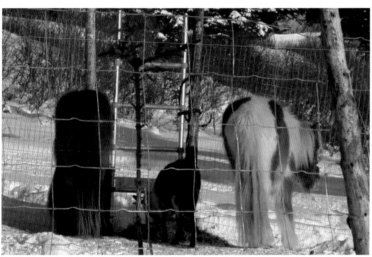

Figure 28
Alvon, Buttercup,
and Hesta

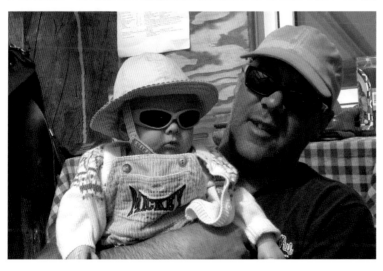

Figure 29
Daddy-daughter
bonding time

Figure 30
Amelia picking
berries

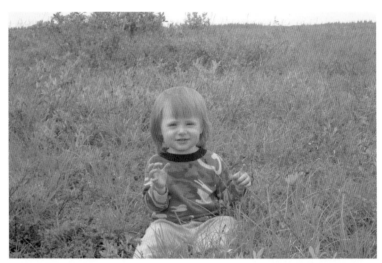

Figure 31
Getting ready for
a boat ride

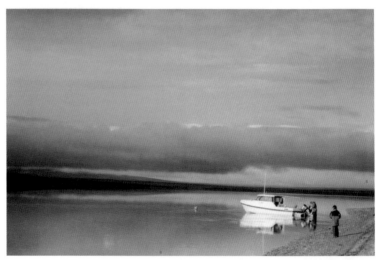

Figure 32
Beachcombing
with Amelia

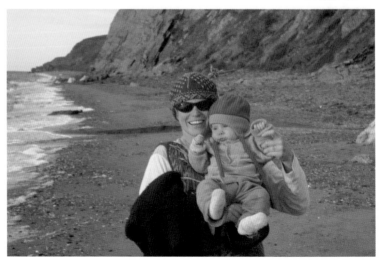

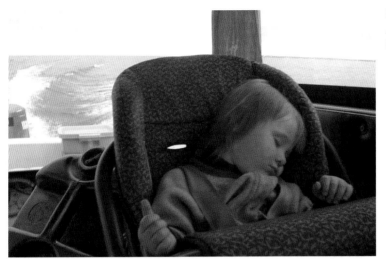

Figure 33
Amelia napping in
her boat seat

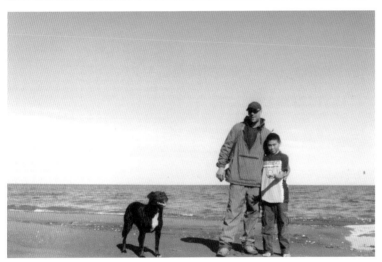

Figure 34
Dave, Alan, and
Penny on the
beaches of Cape
Espenberg

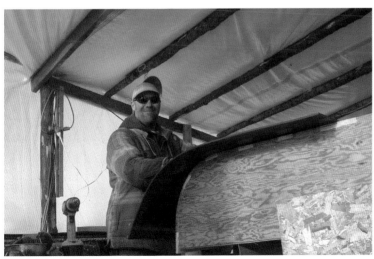

Figure 35
Dave's final
airboat project

Figure 36
The crosses of
Dave and Madi

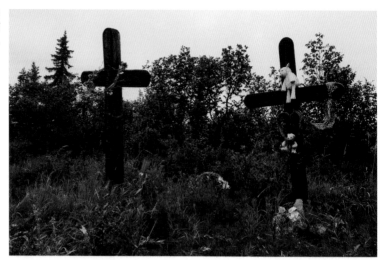

Figure 37
A friend helps
to cut wood

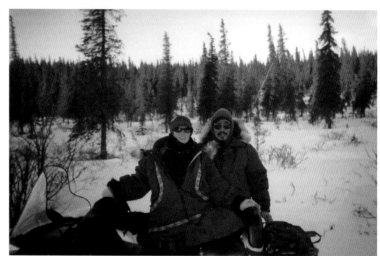

Figure 38
Packing Amelia
on my back for
winter travel

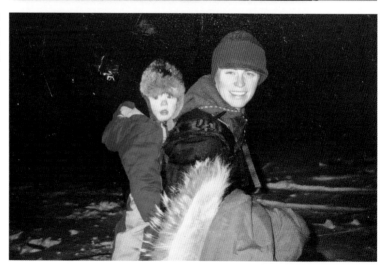

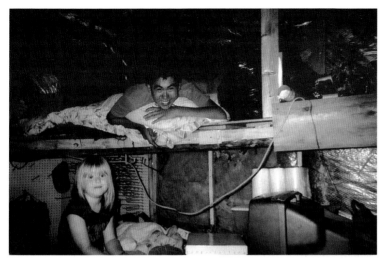

Figure 39
Amelia and Alan
hanging out
at camp

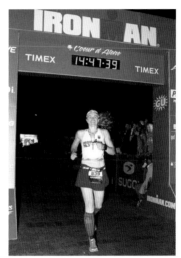

Figure 40
Finishing Ironman
Coeur d'Alene

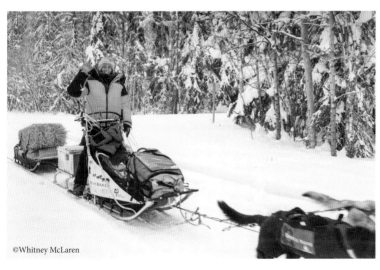

Figure 41
Sled loaded
for the Yukon
Quest

©Whitney McLaren

Figure 42
The finish line of
the Yukon Quest

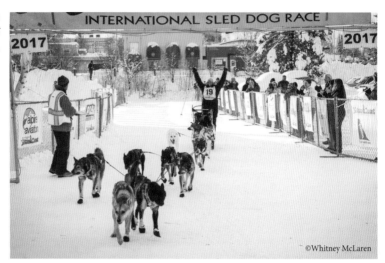

©Whitney McLaren

Figure 43
Amelia and me
hiking up to camp

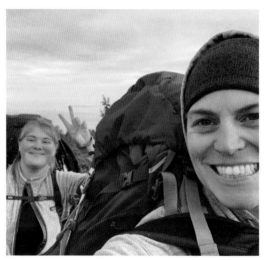

Figure 44
Amelia meeting
me at the end
of the Iditarod

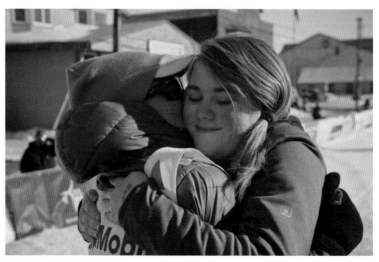

saw and building things. I don't have the technical skill, but work ethic gets me through. I try to build a chicken coop, doghouses, outhouse, greenhouse, etc. It is still so early, but with each passing day, my heart falls deeper in love with Dave. I'm done looking back or even too far forward.

I look up at the sky. "What future is there for Dave and me?" I ask the moon, lacking other company. "How can I help Alan adjust better to life with me? Will I ever not feel so alone? … The nightmares have gone away since moving in with Dave. Are they gone for good now? … Is it okay to want a family? to put down roots in this world?" The moon appears serene and all-knowing, and I hope for answers as if it were an oracle goddess.

The moon answers me the same way she has answered women throughout the eons. Regardless of my words, the moon reaches into my soul and answers the question in my heart, not those in my mind.

"Follow the moon shadow," I hear. "When the heart follows the moon shadow, you will never go astray."

Unsure about the relevancy of the moon's reply, I assume I should follow my heart and look to nature for answers.

Without nightmares plaguing me, my waking hours are relaxed, carefree, and happy. Feeling safe with Dave has positive effects. I tell Dave everything that happened in my past, trusting him to hold my truth and not run away. The struggles that drove me to Alaska slip away from my awareness like a cloud gliding off a mountain top.

The stool Dave carved my name into sits on the side of the house facing east so I can enjoy the incomparable hillside vista. The quiet majesty of the land strikes a healing cord, soothing pains from the past and washing away impurities. The snow sparkles with twinkling fairy dust, a crystal finer than an empress's best, reflecting the sun's warmth in speckled harmony. My mind is as still as the ice which I gaze out upon this clear springlike day in mid-February. The chickadees and blue jays are flocking about, singing and dancing in the richness of the day. The branches of the alder trees wear hoarfrost and look as if they'd grown thorns overnight. Kobuk Lake wears many faces. The glare ice can be as smooth as a baby's bottom or rough and pockmarked like the face of an old man, some areas are riddled with cracks and wrinkles that look like the weathered eyes of a grandmother, and the lake can have large rolling drifts like a giant field of marshmallows.

Building a house and supplying it with gas requires cash. We have a wide variety of entrepreneurial ideas. Local stores overcharge for rifles and ammunition is expensive, so I obtain a federal firearms license. Other than the two stores, there is only one other license holder in town. We order in bulk and help provide local hunters with affordable caribou meat. I dream about opening a bakery in town and calling it Simply Scrumptious. But saving up for a big dream kitchen, I instead stick with bake sales, coffee shop stands, and special orders. Alan has a snow cone machine he sets up at the local softball field. It is a slick appliance that requires a steady supply of ice—tricky without a freezer. Alan becomes an expert at taste-testing different snow cone flavors (see fig. 16).

Dave and I also make money by searching out and selling mastodon teeth, mammoth ivory, and other rarities. The permafrost preserves the remains of these massive, powerful animals that once called northwestern Alaska home. Dave, Alan, and I take off for a week or two at a time in our boat, an Olympic cabin cruiser, to search along the beach bluffs of Kotzebue Sound for long tusks that have fallen out of frozen mud or stick out along the bottoms of rivers. We fill up a couple drums of gas, load them on the boat, grab a tote of food, lots of bug spray, and take off. At night we crawl into the front of the boat to sleep. Good quality mammoth ivory sells for about $130 a pound, so if we uncover a big beautiful tusk, all fossilized, we can sell it for $13,000 to $18,000. Our explorations lead to the discovery of other things that appeal to my archaeological interests as well: ivory carvings, dogsled parts made from bone, glass fishing floats, and other amazing artifacts (see fig. 17).

In the winter, we set gill nets under the ice for sheefish. Dave has a superb system where he catches a bunch of fish, charters a small airplane, then delivers the fish to surrounding villages, where he can trade them for phenomenal carvings he then sells in various stores in Seattle or Anchorage. Dave also makes money as a mechanic, fixing up four-wheelers, snow machines, and outboard motors (see fig. 18).

In our spare time, we build our log cabin by hand, with only the simplest of tools. We dig into a hillside overlooking Kobuk Lake, six hundred yards off the beach. By building into the hill, Dave hopes to keep the north winds from cutting through the house in the winter. Since the hill is all permafrost, digging out the foundation by hand with no excavator has taken two full summers. The sun can melt about two inches of permafrost a day, so we can only dig down that far before having to stop and wait for tomorrow's few inches to thaw. Building a house in the city can be a challenging undertaking. Building a log cabin eighteen miles from town, off the road system, and five hundred miles from the nearest Home Depot, is a different matter altogether (see fig. 19).

In the summer, Dave goes on a trip back home to Washington State to take care of some family business. Alan and I stay at camp watching over things. We drive Dave to the airport with our boat, then go back out to camp after stocking up on groceries for the week. I park the boat in front of our house because the water is too low to make it into the protected lagoon.

The next day a strong storm kicks up from the south with fifty-mile-per-hour winds, and the water level rises. Alan and I nickname it Hurricane Sunflower because it causes all of our sunflowers to fall over. Our boat heaves on the swells, and every passing wave threatens to pull the front anchor out, pushing it closer into shore. I need to move the boat and get it to safety, but I am by myself. I get on my hip boots and take the four-wheeler down to the boat. The water is high, and the four-wheeler is half underwater when the waves come.

I can't both make it to the boat and stay dry. With conviction, I grab the shore anchor and pull the boat in as close as possible. I walk out to it, water going over my hip boots, and make it to the outboard in chest-deep cold water. I heave myself onto the outboard, kicking my knee up onto the lower unit so I can get into the boat. I toss the shore anchor into the boat and now need to start the outboard and pull up the front anchor tied to an eyebolt on the bow. The rocking and heaving is extreme, so my footing is precarious under the wave conditions. Mud and pressure act like cement on the front anchor. I cannot pull it loose.

I start the outboard and get it warmed up so that once the boat is free, I can take off before getting pushed into the beach. For half an hour, I try to free the front anchor. I tie the front anchor to a clip on the boat rail and give the outboard full power to pop the anchor free from the mud. Unsuccessful, I crawl onto the front of the boat and, taking out my knife, cut the front anchor rope, hoping that I can recover it after the storm. I scurry back to the steering wheel and shove the throttle forward, away from the shore. Water pours into the boat until I can angle it into the waves. I steer the boat toward a narrow opening of the lagoon leading to the boat harbor and hope I can make it there without getting pushed up onto the shallow sand bars.

I navigate into the boat harbor. The waves disappear, leaving me to contend only with the wind. After a few breaths, I maneuver to the beach, where I tie off to a permanent anchor. Finding the four-wheeler, I drive back up to the house to check on Alan, sit down by the woodstove, dry off, and enjoy a hot cup of coffee.

Life is full of simple wonders, from the blowing snow to the chickadees. The little, unimportant details just slip away like a hot breath on a chilly night. I learn profound lessons intermingled with the practicalities required by daily life. If we seek answers, solutions are available all around us, clear as day. The richness of living dwells in simple present moments. Why waste it on worries and fears? How can I capture these happy years like fireflies bottled on a hot summer night?

▶IDITAROD, MILE 263
FAREWELL BURN, ALASKA | 2014

You're never the same after you run the Iditarod, and I still
lust to go out and run with dogs, even though I know that I
shouldn't. But I'd give just about anything to be able to do it
again. To see the horizon again from the back of a dog team
would be wonderful.

—GARY PAULSEN

I clear my head and examine the sled. The brush brow gained a hearty
crack from the trip through the Dalzell Gorge and now has failed. This
last tree claims victory by inserting itself through the brow, between the
runners, and down through the base of my sled, which refuses to separate
from it. The dogs want to pull forward; the problem is that the sled needs
go backward about three feet. When brute force fails to move the sled,
I transfer the gang line to the victorious tree, using spare rope to tie the
dogs off to it.

I try to pull the sled free, when Jake Berkowitz comes by. "See? Told
you," he hollers out while putting his hook on a nearby tree to stop his
team. After ensuring they are under control, he walks back and helps pull
my sled off the tree.

"Thanks," I say, depressed. I am in serious risk of not finishing my first
Iditarod. The tree has totaled my sled.

"Have tools?" he asks.

"Yep! I carry about ten pounds of tools and spare parts. I'm good. Thanks for the help."

"Anytime!" Jake shouts as he runs back to his team.

I have no clue what repairs I can make out here that would allow me to go another mile, let alone the fifty to Nikolai. The sled will fall to pieces the next time I hit a stump or rock. To make matters worse, the removable plastic runners that let it glide over the snow wore down in the gorge. In fact, the rocks ripped one of them off, and I have no spares. I am running on aluminum. Using wire, I tie the sled up as best I can. I try multiple configurations, but no matter what I do, there is always a piece of plastic from the bottom of the sled grinding into the dirt and creating drag. After my poor fifteen-minute repair job, I transfer the gang line from the tree back to the sled.

"Ready?" I call to the resting dogs. "Up! Up! *Up!*," I say, hoping we make it a few feet.

A hundred feet later, my fix-it-up job fails. I find another tree to tie off to and get more serious with my sled repair. Duct tape, ripcord, zip ties, and wire find themselves woven into an intricate spiderweb around the runners and sled bottom. I try again, this time with more success. Mile after painstaking mile, we make our way closer to Nikolai. But there's no way we are going to reach it. I think up contingency plans in case the sled falls apart. I could walk the entire way, nursing my sled into Nikolai. Fifty miles at two miles per hour? I could be there in a day.

Two miles after my major crash, I come across Jake, now in the same situation as me. He crashed, and his sled is far beyond repair.

I stop. "Jake, what do you need?"

"Nothing at all. Our race is over."

I am stunned. "What do you mean? Do you need tools?"

"No. I have everything, but the runner and stanchion have both snapped in half. I can't fix this. Just keep going while you still can. I'll figure something out." Jake, a veteran, knows what he is talking about.

The Farewell Burn has seemingly endless numbers of steep hills with sand on the uphill sides and snow only on the downhills—go figure. I stop a dozen times to piece together the sled. We make it into Nikolai eleven hours after leaving Rohn.

At the Nikolai checkpoint, I search for another sled. Martin Buser comes to my rescue and offers me his spare.

"It's not much," he says in his humble manner.

I check out his perfect, homemade, all-plastic sled. "Whatever, this is gorgeous!" I switch my gear over, and my day turns around 180 degrees.

The sled effort takes so much time that the team has slept and is now ready to depart Nikolai. I still have not slept, myself, but the next rest stop is Takotna, where I will take the mandatory twenty-four-hour rest. Sleep for me and food for the dogs will hit the reset button.

Takotna creates a space out of reality to focus on dog care. The dogs are walked to test for stiffness and stretch muscles. To cook their meals, I add four bottles of Heet to the cooker, light it, and then add water or snow to the dog pot along with about ten pounds of chipped fish. These dogs love cooked sheefish, caught and chipped in Kotzebue. I add chipped beef to the cooking fish, then add eight pounds of commercial dog food. This delicious soup takes about twenty minutes to prepare but is worth the wait. I doze in and out of sleep, waking to care for the dogs and feed myself before sleeping more.

After the twenty-four-hour break, the next seven hundred miles follow a predictable pattern of unpredictable trials and triumphs. We travel over rock, sand, tundra, and glare ice out of Unalakleet and over the Blueberry Hills until we find ourselves stuck in a shelter cabin halfway between Shaktoolik and Koyuk for eighteen hours.

▸BREAK-UP

KOBUK LAKE, ALASKA | 2001

Only two things are infinite, the universe and human
stupidity, and I'm not sure about the former.

—ALBERT EINSTEIN

We begin mornings with coffee and toast on the woodstove, listening
to KOTZ Radio to hear the news from around the world. We sit and
talk about our plan for the day. Alan, being a kid, sleeps in as long as
possible. This quiet time starts the day off with a sense of well-being
and connection that keeps us centered. Once awake, Alan drinks hot
cocoa and works on school. Dave goes to "write a letter to the president,"
which is code for using the outhouse. The outhouse view is spectacular.
Overlooking Kobuk Lake, the lights of Kotzebue bubble up to a dome.
In early morning, I keep the door open to admire how the stars glitter
in sync with hoarfrost on tree branches. On lucky days, the northern
lights enter the moment and leave their lasting mark in my mind before
vanishing just as quickly.

Trouble seems so out of place here in the Arctic, where one person is
just a minuscule object when compared to the vastness of the landscape.
The suffering, confusion, and pain rise and then, like the northern lights,
vanish from my sky. I settle into this life and trust it is possible to find
happiness. I yearn for a baby. I am ready and eager to grow the family

with Dave and Alan. With much work to accomplish, however, it is not a convenient time to have a baby.

Life flies by from one season to the next—break-up, summer, freeze-up, long winter. I consider the first day of spring to be December 21, when we gain light by the minute. Summer starts after the last of the ice flows away. The first day of fall is June 21, the longest day of the year. Break-up is one of the most marvelous things to witness. Unable to go anywhere by boat, snow machine, or airplane access, we enjoy our peace. This lasts for two weeks in June. The snow melts and is heavier on the surface and drier and lighter below. These conditions make it easy to punch through the rigid surface up to your hip.

Twenty-four hours of daylight puts life in full swing. The sky and ponds are full of migratory birds. Our schedule adjusts with the changing light. We stay awake until two in the morning and sleep until ten. There are chores to do as we clean up the residue of winter, prevent flooding from snow melt, and provide animal care. Frozen food hides under insulating sawdust. Our increasing number of sled dogs stash food in hidden places that smell awful without snow cover. March seedlings need room to expand to flourish in the greenhouse.

I walk down our beach to the lagoon, where I can witness the daily changes in the ice. Ice separates from the lake floor, which has overflow and ice melt on top of it. The ice breaks away in pieces before a mass exodus of ice sheets make their way out of Kobuk Lake and into the Chukchi Sea.

We are eager to get to town after break-up because after a month with no refrigeration, we are out of cheese, milk, and other supplies. By necessity, the boat was out of the water and high on the gravel beach before the lake froze up in October. Without a truck and trailer, considerable thought and effort goes into the process of putting it back in the water. We use our four-wheeler and an intricate system of tripods, block and tackle, come-alongs, PVC pipe, and rope that Dave rigs together. We work for hours to get the heavy deep-V-bottom boat back in the water. Dave gets the outboard running, replaces the gear oil, and changes out the spark plugs.

We and our neighbor Phillip all hop into the cabin cruiser and head to town. The lake looks clear of ice, but we are unsure of what the jams closer to Kotzebue are like.

"Let's gear up," Dave says.

It is easy to forget what you need on a boat. We should stock it with emergency gear, food, oil, tools, radios, etc. Instead, in a disorderly fashion, we grab a thermos of coffee, life jackets, and a few snacks. Throwing on our hip boots, we drive the four-wheeler down to the lagoon, load up the boat, and take off. The water remains free of ice for eight miles until we approach Lockhart Point on the Baldwin Peninsula. Lockhart Point is the landmark to sight the way to town. The land rises high above the water, visible in all but the foggiest weather or blizzards. Fast-flowing sheets of three-foot-thick ice fill a deepwater channel near Lockhart point. Dave shuts off the engine. Delicate but loud sounds carry out to us—ice chunks bouncing off each other. We deliberate about pressing forward versus going back to camp, but thoughts of the Empress Restaurant's breaded pepper chicken and a chocolate milkshake persuade us to continue on to town.

Phillip ate fatty duck soup last night, gifting him with diarrhea. On a small boat full of people, what do you do? Phillip leans out over the back of the boat's engine mount to take care of business. He needs to make it to town for obvious reasons. Plus, he is out of cigarettes.

We drive along the edge of the channel, waiting for an opening. Ten minutes later, we observe a sparse section. Dave gets the boat moving fast to beat large, oncoming chunks of ice. The risk is getting marooned in the ice floe. If that happens, you can't get free and can damage the boat. After a mile, the ice closes in around us. We're unable to escape. Phillip, again desperate, jumps out of the boat onto a stable sheet of solid ice and pulls his pants down. Hoping to dislodge from the ice, we wait for a couple of hours. As the ice moves downstream, we edge closer to town at less than half a mile per hour. Hours pass by, and we wish we had brought more food. We can all but smell the breaded pepper chicken and french fries from Empress.

Ice grinds the sides of our boat to produce an unnerving screech. Can the ice puncture our fiberglass boat, causing us to take on water? A substantial chunk of ice flips over, slams into the outboard's lower unit, and wreaks permanent damage. Being stranded among three-foot ice blocks is less than ideal. Time to take some serious action.

The radio, forgotten, remains at home. The ice jam thrusts us toward the beach between Lockhart Point and Kotzebue. The compressed ice between us and the beach offers a potential solution.

"I bet you guys could just walk into town," Dave says.

Arching my eyebrows, I stare at him.

"Oh yeah, I do that all the time," Phillip says.

"It's an eight-mile walk. Could be days before I arrive on the boat," Dave says.

I shake my head. "No way. You would be a sitting duck. What can you do for the boat? The ice shows no mercy."

A full-body life jacket, a.k.a. float suit, is in the cabin as a precaution in case the boat springs a leak.

Dave holds up a long wooden pole to push away the ice and grins, "Us cavemen can do a lot with simple tools. Get to town before the opportunity disappears. I'll be fine. Talk to Dickie. He'll know what to do."

Our friend from Kotzebue, Dickie Moto, always seems to know what to do. Phillip is the first to jump out of the boat onto the ice floe. Not wanting to swim, Alan and I dance from one iceberg to the other. Growing up at camp makes Alan a tough kid. He takes large leaps in stride and runs ahead of me. An hour later, we make it to the beach.

Alan fist-pumps the air. "Yeah! We did it!"

Phillip searches for a bush.

Looking back at the boat, Dave seems so far away now, trapped in the ice. While Dave can handle any situation, much of this one is out of his control. We start the eight-mile-long trek into town.

Three hours later, we get to Dickie's house and plan. Dave needs access to food, water, extra clothes, and a VHF radio. An airplane flies over to drop off a float bag of gear. Alan and I stay in town while Dave drifts along with the slow-moving ice. Two days later, and still stuck, Dave passes by on parade before the entire town. Another boat, in the same predicament, joins him. The two boats become the talk of the town. Dozens of people on Shore Avenue with cameras and binoculars point their fingers at the spectacle. Dave seems safe, and I talk to him every few hours on the VHF. The boat's outboard has minor damage but nothing more.

Ice travels in front of town before making its way to the deep water of Kotzebue Sound, where it dissipates. Dave finally gets clear after being stuck on the boat for over fifty hours. Once free, a search-and-rescue boat gets him and tows the boat in. Together, we enjoy our breaded pepper chicken and chocolate milkshakes after the longest trip to town on record. On our way home, I tell Dave the real reason I wanted to go to town. A visit to the hospital has confirmed my hunch: I am pregnant.

▸WOOD

KOBUK LAKE, ALASKA | 2002

Before enlightenment, chopping wood and carrying water.
After enlightenment, chopping wood and carrying water.

—HSIN HSIN MING

Freeze-up lasts from mid-October to mid-November. The summer birds migrate south, and the hours divide themselves equally between the day and night. This is prime caribou-hunting season because we can hang the meat up outside. It freezes by itself, and there are no flies or mosquitoes. I prefer the quiet of winter to the high-energy busyness of summer. Winters are still and filled with a comforting darkness that surrounds you, wrapping you in its embrace. The stars, the northern lights, and the full moon circling the sky provide a mystical backdrop to outdoor activities.

Dave has an Alpine snow machine with two tracks that make it perfect for moving around in the deep snow of the hills. When we travel in our backyard, there are no trails; we make our own. This is easier said than done when the snow is over six feet deep. The Alpine can break trail on steep slopes while maneuvering around logs, stumps, trees, and everything else. It's an impressive piece of machinery.

Dave takes the Alpine, while Alan and I take the Ski-Doo. Both machines pull durable wood flat sleds built by Dave for hauling logs. The Alpine pulls two of them, one long and one short. This combination allows him to carry logs over twenty feet long, which we need for the house. House logs must be large, round, and straight. Alan and I carry the smaller logs for firewood.

After making it to the base of the steep hills at the woodlot, Alan and I wait at the bottom so that Dave can climb into the hills to look for the next section of timber. Dave finds a gully high in the hills that other folks, looking for firewood, tend not to access. The code of the North dictates you don't pilfer someone else's woodlot.

We spend days back in the woodlot. Dave and I have chain saws while Alan picks up branches and moves logs out of the way. My experience felling trees, being none, requires that I learn on the job. Dave is extremely skilled at logging and has no problems going for large trees over two feet in diameter. Our harvested trees are old, dry, and dead, so we won't have to wait years for the curing process.

I get the snow machine stuck in snow at least a couple of times during the day. Alan and I, using a shovel, dig it out to the best of our ability—humbling. Dave doesn't even need the Alpine to pull it out. He knows how to do it and makes me appreciate his skill.

After working for a couple of hours, we start a fire. Spruce twigs and needles serve as kindling. They sound like Rice Krispies, and smell heavenly. We roll logs around the fire, sit down, take a break, and warm our hands by the fire. Thermoses of coffee, hot chocolate, and plenty of food allow us to stay out over long days. I bring dried caribou, salmon, sheefish jerky, trail mix, and sandwiches made on homemade bread. We tease Alan as we laugh and cool off from the sweaty work. The woodlot silence permeates our small group. Branches creak and groan in the wind. Even in winter, birds find a reason to sing.

We tie up our load down at the creek bottom. Getting home, we off-load the logs into piles. Dave has piles set up for the roof section, wall, and foundation. For the sides of the house, logs need to be at least eight inches in diameter. The foundation logs and support logs need to be over a foot in diameter. It takes the three of us to move massive logs around. Leverage and creative thinking benefit us as we shimmy the logs onto piles. My protruding belly reduces my ability to help with this part.

I can use my "plus one" weight for leverage but am not much help when it comes to pushing or pulling. The firewood gets thrown in a different pile. I chainsaw the logs into eighteen-inch-long pieces for the woodstove (see fig. 20).

Dave hoists all the logs with block-and-tackle-style rigging or brute strength. This becomes interesting when putting the logs on the roof. We build the house in a semicircular pattern with the round walls facing the south to mirror the curvature of the beach and to allow for maximum solar exposure during the winter. The house is forty feet long by twenty-five feet wide with one story. Dave manages this with the creative grace of an artist.

▸OUR LITTLEST ANGEL

KOBUK LAKE, ALASKA | 2002

She needs wide open spaces
Room to make her big mistakes.

—DIXIE CHICKS, "WIDE OPEN SPACES"

Up to seven months pregnant, I practice yoga, standing on my head daily. It is hard to no longer act like "one of the guys." I can't drink coffee or whiskey or go out on rough boat rides. I don't quite enjoy being pregnant, despite my excitement about being a mom. Worse than that is being subjected to the impracticality of maternity clothes. I should write to Carhartt and ask them to launch a line of maternity work gear. Those flimsy stretch leggings paired with one of those awful, butt-covering, cutesy dress shirts will not cut it while fishing for salmon, building a greenhouse, or working in the woodlot. Pregnant Alaskans work and need the comfort and practicality of durable gear.

We find out that our baby is a little underweight as she nears full term. I go to Anchorage for the four weeks leading up to her birth. While not on full bed rest, I receive a definite calm-down order. We decide it will be better to give birth in Anchorage, where we have access to the neonatal intensive care unit (NICU), just in case. Anchorage doctors induce a couple of weeks early.

Dave makes it down to Anchorage to be there for the delivery. My mom and thirteen-year-old sister, Cindy, come to be a part of this miracle. On February 28, 2001, we meet our tiny daughter with her shock of red hair. Madilyn Maxine Mackenzie Keith. We call her Madi for short. The doctors discover that she has a hole in her lung, a pneumothorax. She spends two days in the NICU until the hole heals and she has a full lung capacity. I am a new mother, full of naive love and blissful unawareness that anything can ever go wrong.

Madi soon is healthy enough to leave the hospital. Dave and I plan to take Madi home to Kotzebue, but since her birth coincides with the starting week of the Iditarod, we drive my mom and Cindy to downtown Anchorage to watch the dogsled teams go by while I cradle newborn Madi swaddled in cozy knit blankets. I wave at two Kotzebue mushers, Ed Iten and John Baker, and wish them both good luck down the trail. I appreciate their part in the Last Great Race and Madi's first great day.

Dave, Cindy, Madi, and I arrive in Kotzebue still in full-on winter mode and need to travel by snow machine to get home. After stopping first at a friend's house to get a parka large enough to allow me to hold Madi in my arms inside it, Dave drives us home.

Dave loves spending time with Madi. The first month revolves around celebrating her arrival, learning how to be a mother, and trying to get sleep. It is also a time to learn how to balance the demands of hard physical work with fierce protection of this fragile new life. Living out at camp is demanding. There is no running water and no constant source of electricity. There aren't any cars or car seats to put your baby in, no Wal-Mart when you run out of diapers, and no doctors when your baby has a fever. There are no new mom groups and no play dates. No internet exists to look up answers. The phone connectivity is minimal—a party line, meaning anyone can pick up the phone and hear what you're saying. If you want to visit with anyone, it means taking a snow machine or boat into town, which also means putting your newborn baby in a risky situation.

To entertain Madi, and ourselves, we have two dozen chickens. Dave built a nesting box for them outside a window close to the woodstove so they can enjoy the heat. Watching the chickens vie for the best spot and slip off their pegs when they fall asleep is far better than any TV sitcom for a good laugh.

I am accustomed to having the freedom to choose what I want to do next, which is no longer possible with a baby. Boo-hoo, right? The pressures of chores and work wears on me. I can't stand watching Dave do all the hard work, despite his insistence on doing so. The transition is difficult for me. Sitting around the house waiting for a baby to wake up from a nap challenges my way of thinking. For all the inconveniences, the rewards of the peaceful lifestyle and of bringing our kids up in an alternative lifestyle keep Dave and me eager for the future.

While Madi is little, Dave's nephew Dean comes up to help, along with Cindy. Cindy is still in school and has homeschooling to keep current. My dream is to keep her until summer. We all fall in love with this little girl: Madi brings light wherever she goes. Her favorite pastime is to suck on the long beak of a little loon doll given by Grandma to remind her of the fact she has 50 percent Minnesotan in her. This loon becomes a second pacifier to her when she needs help to sleep. Madi sleeps in the bed between Dave and me while Dave works on hand-carving her crib. Our remote camp offers plenty of arms to hold her.

▶ IDITAROD, MILE 795

KOYUK, ALASKA | 2014

I just pulled out of Safety
And I'm on the trail alone
I'm doin' fine and I'm pickin' up time
And headin' on in to Nome.
There's no sled tracks in front of me
And no one's on my tail
I did, I did, I did the Iditarod Trail!

—HOBO JIM, "THE IDITAROD TRAIL SONG"

The dogs and I are stuck at the Shaktoolik shelter cabin for eighteen hours. Freezing and hungry, we cannot delay any longer. We make our way, trail stake by trail stake, for the next thirty-five miles. I arrive in Koyuk shaken up but surrounded by curious school kids asking questions and wanting my autograph. One special young girl helps put out straw for the dogs. Her eager attitude cheers me and helps me realize that I have to suck it up and keep my head in the game. The dogs look solid, feel great, and are eating well. The storm was harder on me than them. There is still a race going on.

The trail from Koyuk to Elim is beautiful, hard, and fast most of the way except for the new snow drifts. We leave at night, the dogs' favorite time to run. My team is the first out of Elim and takes the burden of breaking out the trail. After ten miles, the faster teams behind me catch up and break out the remaining trail.

The trail from Elim to White Mountain is difficult—history paints a picture of mushers and teams breaking down—not only for the large amount of hill climbing but also for crossing sea ice between Golovin and White Mountain. The intense climbing makes the views all the more rewarding. The final summit is one thousand feet up to the height of Little McKinley. There is no wind the day I cross Golovin Bay, so the glare ice poses no threat as the team is able to maintain adequate traction without the complicating sideways force of wind.

At White Mountain everyone takes an eight-hour mandatory rest before tackling the remaining seventy-seven miles of trail to Nome. The trail to Safety requires yet more climbing up through the Topcock Hills. After the summit, the trail drops for two miles to the coast. There is little snow on this descent again and my sled brake gives out. I careen down steep, rocky side slopes with an excited dog team and no way to slow them down. I stop a couple times by giving commands to the dogs and tip my sled over to wire the brake together. Dropping to the coast, we move north through the "Blowhole." Conditions deteriorate to ten-foot visibility with the wind blowing forty miles per hour. The dogs need to cross glare ice with sand and snow drifts. The wind blows the sled sideways into tripods and tree stumps and anything else in between. Close to Nome, we still have many obstacles to overcome. The dogs do the best they can, and we make painstaking progress.

The checkpoint of Safety is twenty-two miles outside Nome and a scary point for mushers. The dogs recognize the roadhouse as a checkpoint and are eager to investigate the straw and happy vets. People often come out to cheer the teams on, and the dogs would like to join the party. I need to drop a dog, Heineken, who has a sore wrist. The remaining dogs think this is a great place to hang out for a while to escape the storm. Three hundred feet past the checkpoint, the dogs decide that instead of their usual seven-and-a-half-mile-per-hour pace, they want to go four and a half miles per hour. If only they knew we are less than three hours from the end.

I stop to consider the situation. By consider, I mean I sit on my sled to cry out loud for a good ten minutes. After my pity party is complete, I switch around the dogs and put in new leaders. Even if I have to push the sled the whole way, it is better than sitting on the sled crying like a baby in the middle of a snowstorm. four and a half miles per hour is what we do all the way to Nome. I kick, run, and pole with everything I have left (see fig. 21).

People drive out on the roads to cheer the team on. The dogs and I feel the excitement building. We drop onto the sea ice and the siren blows to welcome the next dog team to Nome.

The trail goes up a small hill to the front street of Nome where fans holler out "Good Job!" and "Congratulations!"

We are the thirty-second team into Nome, but I feel like a champion. The Burled Arch, marking the finish line since 1975, beckons us in, where a crowd awaits. Amelia, my daughter, is there, waiting to ride on the sled with me to the finish line (see fig. 22).

My mom is there crying with relief. I tell her not to cry because then I will. This is a total celebration. We made it. I relish the sheer feeling of accomplishment that comes from making it 1,049 miles to Nome despite the exhaustion, frustration, and disappointment we had along the trail.

"I did, I did, I did, the Iditarod Trail!" Hobo Jim's lyrics come back to me.

We park the team in the dog lot. It feels like a piece of me is taken away as I watch them go, knowing our great adventure together is at an end. Eight out of fourteen dogs finish the race. Summit, Ears, Joy, Neo, Huffy, Ghoulie, Papa, and Lightening all deserve medals. Summit and Ears led together for 90 percent of the race. They did an incredible job keeping us safe and on the trail. Knowing the dogs are being cared for, I go to a hotel room; take a long, hot shower; eat a delicious meal; and enjoy the company of family and friends. After a few days of sleep, I am now restless. I look outside at the clear, sunny day and recall the gorgeous days climbing through the Alaska Range and when I first came in to Unalakleet to see the ocean coast. I dream about the next adventure.

▶HELPLESS

KOBUK LAKE, ALASKA | 2002

Love is the strongest and most
fragile thing we have in life.

—VANESSA PARADIS

It is a morning like many others. The house is cold and quiet after shutting down the woodstove so the fire wouldn't die overnight. Dave and I lie together on the outer half of the bed, giving the inner half, boxed in by the wall, to Madi. Madi stirs after waking up twice that night. Dave jumps up to put wood in the stove and warm the house before we get out of the covers. I prop up pillows against the back wall and cradle Madi in my arms.

"How did you sleep?" I ask Dave.

"Like a baby," he says as he leans over to kiss Madi on top of her fuzzy, red-haired head. "Well, not like our baby."

I nurse Madi while Dave makes coffee. The house feels alive with warmth as the aromas of ground beans and the sounds of crackling firewood fill the air. I am not feeling eager to get out of bed. Dave turns on KOTZ Radio and NPR News tells us about events around the world. As our only source of news, I hang on every word.

Dave comes into the back bedroom. "Are you ladies ready for some toast?"

Deciding that it is worth getting out of bed, I stifle a yawn and respond with a yes that sounds like a mix of yeah, yes, ah, and ugh.

I put on a pair of sealskin slippers that Dave and Alan gave me for Christmas. Changing Madi's diaper takes only a moment. I dress her in warm pajamas and swaddle her in a blanket. Madi and I assume our rocking chair by the woodstove, where I can prop my feet up near its door while holding Madi in my lap.

Dave looks at us. "I think you have the better part of this deal. Maybe I should hold the baby while you put on some toast."

Holding his arms out to Madi, it is clear he wants daddy-daughter time. Happy to oblige, I hand her over. My bladder reminds me of my own needs, so I dress for a trip to the outhouse. I put on sweatpants, a sweatshirt, a camouflage pullover winter jacket, a wool hat, fleece gloves, and my heavy winter boots. Overall, I look like I am attempting a trip to Mars. Outside now, it looks like I *am* on Mars. The early morning is still black, and the cold spring air is harsh as it enters my lungs. The moon is absent from the sky allowing me a full view of close to a zillion stars. Packed snow defines the outhouse path. It needs no door because it faces into a thick grove of trees. Pulling down my pants, I cringe as I know that sitting down on the ice-cold pink foam board is going to not feel super good. Taking a moment to appreciate my surroundings, I allow my body to relax into the natural beauty around me even in this wintry Arctic March morning.

From outside, I hear Dave talking to Madi in a bunch of nonsensical gobbledygook: "Baby googi gagga dadda. Yai ma nee cho to be baby baby baby."

I enter the house smiling, seeing just how much this little baby adores her daddy. Madi laughs as Dave makes funny faces at her. The happy sounds wake up the household. Neither of them is a morning person, but Cindy and Alan's eyes are sparkling as if laughing at some secret joke only they know about.

"Good morning!" I run over to my little sister and give her a big hug. My sister gives the best hugs in the universe, full of unconditional love and strength even at thirteen years old.

Alan, not being in the mood for a hug, assumes a makeshift karate stance. "Try it, I dare ya." I don't dare and cut up slices of bread to heat on a piece of aluminum foil by the woodstove.

"What do you want to do today?" I ask the crowd.

"I'd like to stay right here all day, oh yes I would," Dave says, more to Madi than me. "But … I suppose I need to go to the woodlot. Every day we miss puts us at risk for not getting our house built." Dave senses my worry. "I mean, I should stay focused while we have a good trail to haul logs on and while Dean is here to help. What are you gals going to do?"

"I think we will swing a little, then change a few diapers, feed the baby, hold the baby, and play with the baby," I say, somewhat stuck in the routine of new motherhood.

I am struck with a joyful thought. "What if we grab a load of logs? Cindy, Alan, and I could drive out and bring lunch. We can share a fire and go home," I say, rejuvenated at the thought of being helpful.

Still holding Madi, Dave says, "You do not need to do that. You have a lot on your plate right now."

I insist it is good for us. "Madi hasn't been napping much during the day and has been colicky. Snow machine rides always calm her down."

Cindy wants her turn with Madi and leans down to kiss her cheek. Dave, sensing the need of Auntie Cindy, gives up Madi to her. I pull over her swing. She is big enough today to sit in it and proud of it (see fig. 23).

I turn to Cindy. "Want to go?"

"A trip to the woodlot with a fire sounds refreshing," Cindy replies, and we both agree that it will do Madi good to get out of the house.

"All right," Dave says, overruled. "But if you change your mind, don't worry about it. I have a plan either way."

Dave and Dean gather gear to prepare for the trip out. Alan wants to go. Although he has homework, Dave allows him to come. Hearing this, Alan's mood changes. He would much rather be at the woodlot with his Dad than home with three bossy girls doing schoolwork.

Madi fusses as if knowing her Dad is getting ready to leave. Cindy puts her in the swing, and Madi is somewhat appeased.

"You think she will be okay going to the woodlot?" Cindy asks.

I consider how we will do it. I have a set of oversized insulated coveralls that have perfect suspenders built in with a belt around the waist. I can nestle Madi in the front of me with her swaddling secured between the suspenders and the belt. This keeps her in place and prevents the cold air from getting to her tiny toes and arms.

"I'm sure," I say. "On previous trips into town she relaxes with the motion of the snow machine and falls asleep. She wakes up in a much better mood."

Cindy nods but her eyebrows are knit in consternation. She looks at Madi swinging. "But the trip to town ends in a warm house."

She has a good point. The trip to the woodlot takes about forty-five minutes, and we are about eight miles from any shelter. The ride back will be slower with a loaded sled.

"Can you drive with a load of logs?" I ask. "If Madi is fussy, then I'll need to ride and can't help drive the load of logs back." I am not worried about her ability, because my little sister has driven a snow machine with a sled more than enough times, but I don't want to take anything for granted. I want to feel out her confidence level.

"Yeah, of course," Cindy says without doubt.

We need to help. We can do this.

After a filling breakfast, Dave goes outside to fill the snow machines with gas, oil, and tools and get the sleds connected. Madi cries, and I pick her up from the swing to comfort her. As soon as Dave comes into the house, Madi stops crying.

"How do you do that?" I ask with an exasperated voice tighter than I wanted.

Dave is ready to leave. He does a round of teasing goodbyes. "Baby, be nice to your mama. Cindy, be nice to the baby. Kat, don't worry about coming out if it's too much. I love you."

After Dave shuts the door behind Dean and Alan, Madi cries. She continues crying for the next four hours. Cindy and I try to do everything possible to see to her needs.

"She needs to take a nap but won't sleep," I say. "Let's head to the woodlot. She will calm down."

I try to nurse Madi before we pack up, but she refuses to eat. We begin the long process of assembling our gear, assembling Madi, and assembling food, all while Madi cries at the top of her lungs. I am tense from all the details needing attention.

We leave the yard. I drive knowing my arms, going out to the handles of the snow machine, form a perfect car seat to keep her secure in. The windshield blocks more of the wind for the driver, so Madi is warm. Madi still screams. Her loud yells compete with the roar of the machine. I stop after five minutes to unzip my oversized snowsuit to see if I can make any adjustments, but she is cozy and warm.

"Maybe she'll eat now," I say.

Cindy just shrugs, doing her best to stay positive with the whole situation.

I have my clothing fixed so I can open it and give Madi access to nurse. She does. She goes back and forth between nursing and screaming.

"Maybe if we keep driving, she will settle down," I say. I resume driving, knowing Madi is secure and settling down.

I stop a few minutes later to check on her, and she is now more relaxed and nursing. "We are good!"

Cindy and I high-five each other. We continue. I unzip every few minutes to see if Madi has fallen asleep and make sure her face, hands, and feet are warm. Things look better, and I settle into the enthusiasm of making it to the woodlot.

I need to be useful. After the long months of pregnancy, being in Anchorage for the delivery, and being housebound for the past month, I have felt a massive urge to contribute to all we are working for at home. Being a mother is all I hoped it could be, but I need to be a mother *and* a good team member doing her part. Lost in a moment of reverie, I notice a lack of movement inside my parka.

"Yay! She's napping!" I yell to Cindy. Now she will get caught up on her rest and feel better. I stop the snow machine to check on her positioning again and look down to see her quiet resting face. Relieved that she is resting, I put my hand inside to touch her cheek with love. Then I see it: blood dripping out of her nose.

"Cindy, something is wrong," I say while unzipping my one-piece suit. "Madi, what happened?" I ask as if our baby could talk.

The blood has dripped down her nose and chin to my chest. I try to wake her up. I tap her on her shoulders. "Baby girl, wake up. Madi. Madi. Madi?" She is not responding.

"Cindy, I need to get her out of this coat."

The two us work to extract Madi from her carrier as fast as we can, then lay her on the seat of the snow machine. I don't see or hear her breathing. She is just lying there, still. I search for a pulse but also can't feel anything. It must just be hard to feel in a baby.

Having CPR training, I know this is what I need to do: I lower my head and breathe into her mouth, thinking this will startle her enough to trigger a response. Still nothing. I place my mouth over her tiny nose and mouth and continue in a regular sequence of breaths. We feel again for breathing and a pulse. I look at Cindy, face taut with fear and white with cold and shock. Nothing. I know I need to do compressions with my fingers. Is it my index finger? middle finger? on her sternum or above? I am frantic, crazed. Panic wells up inside, causing my vision to blur. I act: compressions, two breaths, repeat. Still no response. Repeat.

We need help but how? I look around. We are at least four miles from our camp and four from where Dave is in the woodlot. I need him. He will know how to fix her. I have to keep doing CPR. I wonder if Cindy can find him.

"Cindy, do you think you can follow the trail to the woodlot and find Dave? I don't know how far up the hill he is. Look to see what trail looks fresh. Listen for a chain saw. Yell loud—sound carries, and he will hear you." I go back to doing another round of CPR. "Can you unhitch the trailer?"

Cindy nods, relieved to act and look away from the horrific scene in front of her: Madi's blood smeared on my face from the CPR and her lifeless form on the snow machine.

After she separates the trailer, I move Madi onto it. "Cindy, be careful. It's easy to get stuck. Drive as fast as you can, but don't go faster than you can handle. Don't get hurt. Find Dave."

"OK. I got this," Cindy says.

My last words to her send panic rising to top of my throat. As Cindy takes off, nausea forces me to bend down and vomit. No time. I have to keep doing CPR, so I rush back to Madi and continue another series.

"Madi, come on! Madi, come back! Madi, where are you? What happened?" I am screaming now at the top of my lungs. "Madi! Come back!"

Between spurts of CPR I look for signs of help. Nothing but desolate, lonely, useless frozen tundra. The nearest doctor, in Kotzebue, is a twenty-five-mile snow machine ride away. The fear inside me transforms to desperation as my breathing becomes fast and shallow.

Crying now and hysterical, still doing CPR, I say, "Madi, I need you. Come on. I'm so sorry. I'm sorry. Madi, come back. Please! Please!" I plead to God, Buddha, the Great Spirit, everyone, "Don't do this! She is just a baby! Punish me. I don't care. Just don't hurt her. Don't take her away. Don't take my baby! Please. I will do anything. I am sorry for whatever I did. Just don't take her. Don't take her. Please." CPR continues, but no answer comes from the God I beg to. I shake Madi for a response. Nothing.

I continue CPR in a shocked blur, losing all sense of time. Then, I feel arms coming around me. Dave has arrived. Cindy made it. She found him. He is magic and can fix anything.

Dave asks, "What happened?" I continue doing CPR while I explain.

He leans over Madi and feels for a pulse then examines her. "We need to get her home and call for a medic."

He hooks up the trailer to the snow machine so I can keep doing CPR. Cindy stays behind with Dean and Alan to load up the tools and hurry back to the house.

As we drive back home, I worry about the temperature for Madi. I try to estimate the elapsed time in my head. Five minutes before Cindy went to the wood lot. Thirty minutes to get there and back. Five minutes getting sorted out to head home. Madi hasn't breathed for forty minutes. The cold permeates her exposed tiny body. Her fingers feel frozen despite the blankets and coverings. I do my best to keep her covered while doing CPR in the bumpy back of the snow machine trailer. Once we get there, Dave jumps off to help me get up. My body is numb, but we make it with Madi inside the house. Dave picks up the phone to call 911.

He answers their questions. "It has been over an hour. What do we do? It will take us another hour and a half to make it to town doing CPR." He listens then responds, "OK, we will be ready."

Turning he says, "They are bringing out a helicopter. They should be here in twenty minutes. Want me to take over?"

I continue CPR. Maybe I don't know where to find her pulse. If I keep her blood flowing and air moving the medics can revive her. "No, it's okay. I've got it." I need to be doing everything possible to help her.

Dave sits there in a mortified stupor staring at the sky for the first sign of the helicopter. He sees it and rushes out to get the snow machine started. He watches where the helicopter lands. It maneuvers down to the sea ice at the bottom of hill in front of our house. Dave picks up two medics with their gear. They drive up and run into the house. Relief floods through me. I stop CPR because the medics will save her.

They check her airway, breathing, and pulse. Looking at each other, they evaluate the situation. They ask me to describe what happened while they assemble a breathing device with a mask to put over her face. They resume aspirations and tell me they can do nothing more.

One paramedic says, "Madam, we need to get her to town."

Dave helps me switch into different clothes and drives us down to the helicopter. He loads us into the helicopter and tells me he will be right behind on the snow machine. He first needs to ensure the safety of Dean, Cindy, and Alan. The helicopter ride takes an eternity. Mental math continues. One hour and ten minutes to get back to the house, twenty minutes for the medics—a total of one and a half hours. I stare at Madi's face being pumped with air by the medic. Flying back to Kotzebue, we are at two hours—two hours since Madi's pulse kept her alive. Two hours ago, she was screaming, and I wished her to be asleep. It's two and a half hours until we make it to the hospital and the doctors declare the time of death to be 4:13 p.m., March 29, 2002.

A friend, Lena Ferguson, comes to the hospital to sit with me. The doctors let me sit in the emergency room holding Madi while they examine her and ask questions. I don't hear what they are saying but stare at the hospital wall. Lena holds my hand and grips it, asking me if I heard the doctors.

"What?" I ask.

"She will need to stay here with us," one of them says. "We will bring her to Anchorage for an autopsy. You will want to know what happened."

This didn't sink in. I will not leave my baby. She needs me. I grip her in my arms.

"What happened?" I asked them, begging for answers. "What happened to her?"

"I don't know," the doctor says. "These things just happen sometimes. Babies die, and we don't know why. This seems like SIDS which affects babies under six months."

"Was it her lung?"

He looks at me, confused.

"She had a hole in her lung at birth. The hospital said they fixed it. Was it her lung?"

"It's possible. We won't know until they can do that autopsy."

Numbness permeates my head, my chest, my belly.

"Kat, we need to leave Madi with the doctors," Lena says with compassion. "The doctors will care for her." She walks over to get a pair of scissors and finds an envelope. She leans over and cuts off a piece of her red downy hair and puts it in the envelope. "You will want this later," she says, putting it into my coat pocket.

I cling onto Madi unwilling to let go.

Dave walks into the room. "Hey, baby," he says, bending down by me to take a long, heartbreaking look at his baby girl. His eyes are only for his daughter.

Realizing the permanent conclusion of daddy-and-daughter time, I lose control. Understanding of what this means washes over me, burning me like acid. Inside my head, a loud cry of anguish rips open my heart. Horrified and desperate, deep down I know the truth my mind still can't grasp.

Dave looks me in the eyes. "It's time to say goodbye now."

He wants me to give her to the nurse. I look at her wondering who she thinks she is that she can have our baby when we can't. I am physically unable to let her go. Looking down at our Madi, I rub my fingers against her soft cheeks, along the line of her nose, and her lips, I twirl my fingers through her hair and lean down to smell her newborn baby smell. I hug her close, as if I can will her to scream again.

"Scream as loud as you want, Madi. Just wake up," I whisper.

I hand her to Dave so he can say goodbye. He holds her for a moment, leans down, and kisses her. His frozen frame tells me his anguish is threatening to take control. Looking at me, as if lending strength he doesn't have, he hands our baby over to the doctor.

"We will call you when we know something." The doctor takes her and walks out the door.

I stand then crumple to the floor, all of my will to continue now gone.

"Let's go home," Dave says. "Alan and Cindy need us."

Those words remind me we are not alone in this devastation. The kids need us. Another wave of horror, a deep chasm of pain, rips me open knowing what this news will do to them. I cannot talk to friends in the waiting room gathered there for us. The chief of police is there and needs to ask questions. I sit down in a corner chair, unmoving, while Dave talks to the chief and others.

"There wasn't anything we could do. She's gone," I overhear him say. "Thank you for coming. We need to get home."

Dave excuses us, and I follow his lead as we get on our winter gear and head out to where Dave parked the snow machine in front of the emergency room doors.

It is evening now, and the spring sun hides behind a thick grayness of clouds that mirrors our emptiness and despair. My parka is oversized and ill-fitting without Madi in it. How can we leave her there? Who will take care of her? It doesn't seem to make any sense why she isn't with us. The numb hollowness wars with the desperate madness urging me to go back and get her. My breasts harden with milk, painful with every jarring bump of the snow machine. Madi needs to nurse now. She must be hungry. After a long hour we make it home.

Dave walks in first and I follow.

Dave speaks soft and with love, "I am so sorry. She didn't make it."

Cindy breaks down at these words, and I reach over to hold her while she cries. Cindy held hope that the hospital could pull off a miracle. Alan goes quiet and then, stone-faced, hugs his Dad. Alan wants to comfort him. Alan looks at me with a heavy concern no nine-year-old should know. Dean, who was trying to hold it together for the kids, lets a single tear slide down his face. Hours go by, and the five of us sit by the wood-stove staring at the empty swing in the middle of the room where just that morning Madi was contentedly swinging. On the tabletop sits the loon whose little beak comforted her before going to sleep. Everywhere I look there are signs of our little girl. It is impossible to overstate the impact she had on our lives. Agony runs through my soul and sets fire to my painful breasts. I do nothing about it though. This pain is tangible, and if I focus on it, perhaps the death of my soul will be less noticeable.

Part Three

SCRATCHING

▸IDITAROD, MILE 0
FAIRBANKS, ALASKA | 2015

Courage is the power to face difficulties. Courage
comes from a reserve of mind more powerful than outside
circumstances. When we are bigger than our problems,
we gain the courage necessary to win.

**—FROM *THE BEST OF SUCCESS*
BY WYNN DAVIS**

Not everything goes according to plan.

Not even the start of the 2015 Iditarod race goes according to plan this year. Iditarod 2015 begins in Fairbanks because of snow shortages in the Dalzell Gorge. The race committee is not eager to have a repeat of the injuries that defined 2014. The Fairbanks restart keeps everyone, including the race officials, working up new strategies. There is a significant amount of chaos because it has been twelve years since Fairbanks hosted the start (see fig. 24).

After the ceremonial start in Anchorage, all the teams make the 360-mile drive north to Fairbanks. There is a major snowstorm that causes mushers to drive off the road. The drive takes over twelve hours. Teams take off every two minutes from Fairbanks and head toward Nenana. Teams pass back and forth, all going at different speeds. Some sprint to get ahead of the masses. I keep the dogs traveling slow to avoid blowing out any wrists or shoulders. For the first couple of days of the race, nine miles per hour is ideal to get these dogs trail-hardened.

My race plan is to go through Nenana, avoid the confusion of the first checkpoint, and camp ten miles out. The dogs are overexcited. They don't care about resting. The entire team is hyper and wants to play with each other, fight over food, and bark at every single dog team passing by. Not one of us, musher or dog, sleeps.

After a four-hour stop, we travel forty-five miles to camp between Nenana and Manley Hot Springs. At Manley, I drop my main leader, Summit. Summit is the leader every musher hopes for. Everyone knows Summit, not only for his looks but for his loving attitude. He is keen on affection yet royal and aloof in poise and posture. He isn't a fast trotter, and his shoulder aches. I planned on his stable presence to make it to Nome and worry about leaving him behind.

I leave Manley Hot Springs with fifteen dogs and head to Tanana for the remaining fifty-six miles. I carry two dogs in my sled for thirty miles. We rest in Tanana for six hours, and I leave three dogs behind. At Tanana, the trail follows the mighty Yukon River, the longest in Alaska and Yukon. Its surface area is 25 percent that of Texas. Historically, it was a principal means of transportation during the Klondike Gold Rush. It remains a local snow and water highway for villages along the river. The trail from Tanana to Ruby is close to 120 miles, and we camp halfway between Tanana and Ruby on the riverbank of the Yukon.

In contrast to my 2014 rookie Iditarod, I plan on camping outside the checkpoints as much as possible now. I have learned what a unique and fulfilling experience it can be camping out on the Yukon. I start a fire to warm my hands and look up to enjoy a sky full of stars.

Ruby is 396 miles into the race, and I am down to twelve dogs. They are looking bored with the Yukon. Time to change my race strategy. Extended rest may increase speed and prevent further injury from happening. I take my eight-hour mandatory layover in Ruby.

The trail from Ruby to Galena is only fifty miles, but temperatures are now forty-five below zero. Cold air sinks deep into the Yukon River making this a long and dangerous run.

▶CEREMONY

KOBUK LAKE, ALASKA | 2002

I keep a close watch on this heart of mine.

—JOHNNY CASH, "I WALK THE LINE"

Waking up in the cold, dark bed, I know it is in the early hours of the morning. Dave gets up before I do and fires up the woodstove to heat the house. I lean over, putting my arm out, to check on Madi. Panic rises in my throat, cutting off my breathing when I don't find her. The sudden movement flares up pain in my swollen breasts as understanding dawns. Madi is dead. My stomach rolls over as images of blood coming out of her nose flash before me. I jump over Dave trying to reach the slosh bucket, knowing I won't make it outside in time to throw up. I splash cold water over my face trying to clear away the living nightmare. It doesn't work.

"I'm here babe," Dave says—he came out after me. He doesn't ask how I am or tell me everything will be okay. There are no fake platitudes between us. I am here for you. I love you. We are both in a state of constant anguish, but we will navigate our way through this together somehow. We are stronger together than alone.

My mom and Dave's dad come up for the funeral. A synthetic casket isn't right for Madi. All week Dave spends time in his shop working on making one from wood we brought down from the hills earlier in the year. I spend hours trying to come up with a suitable design for the lid. I start one drawing, cry all over the page, rip it up, and start all over. The night before we bury Madi, I stay up to carve a Celtic cross with a spiral at the heart onto the lid (see fig. 25).

Our friend Chuck makes her a cross from black spruce and stains it with linseed oil. Carved into it are the words "Our Littlest Angel." Countless friends come to camp to help with the burial and support us. The ground is permafrost and we need a jackhammer along with many shovels. The box is so tiny. We bury Madi next to our new house, still under construction—the house that she was to grow up in.

We try to discover what happened. Maybe the hole in her lung didn't heal all the way. When her breathing became hard from all the crying she did, perhaps it burst open. The autopsy comes back with results. She died from positional asphyxiation. Her body position in my parka exerted pressure on her lungs so she couldn't breathe. I will live with the unbearable knowledge, shame, and guilt. Gut wrenching sobs of devastation permeate my entire being and take over any control I have of my sanity.

Together, Dave and I get the woodstove fired up and make coffee. Each of us knowing our part of the routine and able to work together without speaking. We look away at the many areas of the house dedicated to our tiny girl. She filled up the house like she filled up our hearts. The comfort of the routine calms down my stomach and throat, allowing me to talk. "Thank you," I say, embracing Dave in a tight hug, as if I am affirming he is real. I feel I wouldn't be able to exist without him. I take a deep breath. "What would you like to do today?"

Dave looks at me with sudden seriousness. "I want to marry you today."

I smile. "I will marry you any day. Are you sure this is the right time?"

"Our families are all up here at camp. Let's honor the memory of our baby. We need to give Alan and our families hope right now. We need to be the strong ones for them."

We have been discussing getting married for months and agree that now is the time to commit to one another. It overjoys our families.

"I love you" is all I can say. "Okay, let's do it. Today is our wedding day then. Are you supposed to even see me?"

Dave just laughs and turns to get his hot cup of coffee.

The house wakes as the sleeping family smells coffee. The sound of crackling firewood and its heat invite people to get out from under their covers. We have family sprawled everywhere.

My mom is first. "Good morning. You two are up early." She gives Dave a hug before her own daughter—a trend that continues.

Trying to keep the mood light I say, "Gee, Ma, he's not even your son-in-law yet, but he's already your favorite."

Mom says, as she always does when so accused, "I love all my kids the same."

She turns and says, "Good morning, kiddo." Hugging me she asks, "How is the pain today?"

I look at her with a big smile on my face and shrug. "No pain today, because it is my wedding day."

My mom knows me well enough. She looks at my eyes to judge my mood not my mouth, which wears a smile even if my eyes are dark and dead. Mom gets ibuprofen and runs right into Dewey, Dave's father.

"Well, good morning," he says in a deep baritone voice. Mom shakes her head, laughs, and continues around him. Dewey comes in. This time, I get the first hug.

I look at Dave in triumph. "At least I am someone's favorite."

Dave shrugs his shoulders and lifts his hands up, feigning innocence. "I got in a lot of trouble as a kid."

"Boy, you got that right. Did he ever!"

Alan pops his head out over the edge of the loft where he slept. "What kind of trouble?" He can't wait to get dirt on his Dad.

"Wouldn't you like to know," Dave says.

Dewey winks to Alan. "If you get on up out of bed, I will tell you all about it."

Alan, with a smile full of mischief, decides it isn't worth it and crawls back under his blanket.

Mom takes advantage of the distraction and slips me ibuprofen knowing I don't want attention on me.

"Thanks, Mom," I whisper, before downing them with coffee.

Alan's momentary exuberance wakes up Cindy sleeping in the loft we call the bat cave. Sleepy-eyed, she looks down and tries to decide if it is worth coming downstairs.

"Morning, Cinderella," Mom calls out using the nickname my sister loves to hate. Without speaking, Cindy comes downstairs and joins us. Her eyes are distant and swollen from crying. Her nightmares mirror my own. I give her a long hug, wishing she didn't have to go through this.

Mom turns to the group after looking outside. "Looks like we have a beautiful day for a wedding."

In early April, the sun rises at seven o'clock. The world comes alive with color, and the brilliant blue sky plans to stick around for the day. Birds are singing from the trees, and the dogs outside are chewing on a new discovery of meat chunks that have thawed out from the intense sunlight. We sit down to breakfast, and I know Dave is right. It delights everyone to have a meaningful goal for the day: a wedding. After a week full of helpless despair, our family needs to do something, fix something, act to control life again.

My mom gets out a pad of paper and pencil. "What needs to happen?"

Dave and I look at each other. I hear none of the conversation as I get lost in his eyes. Our love gives me courage, strength, comfort, and peace. I am used to surviving this world and fixing things by myself. After today, I won't be alone anymore. Dave will be there, and as partners, we can fix things together. I am not a loner anymore. Strange, I don't want to be. I feel more like myself when I am with him than I do alone.

"Katie?" My mom calls me out of my reverie.

Turning away from Dave, I say, "Yeah, Mom? Sorry."

"What time will people be able to come out?"

"One o'clock. Camp teacher will be out here at about eleven"

"Camp teacher" is the nickname we gave our good friend Eric Smith who snow-machines out to different camps and teaches homeschoolers. Later that morning, we see snow machines heading our way. The vantage point of the house enables us to see incoming traffic for miles away, giving us ample warning to expect guests. Eric is the first to arrive.

"Hot off the press!" he says before even taking his gear off. "I am now an ordained minister of the Universal Life Church of Modesto California."

Eric explains to us that the Universal Life Church is a nondenominational religious group that advocates for religious freedom. Their online ordination process allows anyone to become a minister free of charge. "Nothing to it," he says and grins. His long black hair falls over his camouflage jacket as he pulls his cigarettes from his ripped jeans and hands one to my Mom. The juxtaposition of appearances illustrates the unique individual that is "camp teacher" Eric.

Others soon arrive after hearing radio announcements of the upcoming ceremony. Sandra Moto helps my mom and Cindy bake a wedding cake. Sandra and her husband, Dickie, have come every day during the past week. Good friends are scarce, but when times get tough, they stay without being asked.

While the cooking is happening, Dave and I fade in and out of the craziness. We clean up and dress. Showering is not simple with so many people, no running water, and no privacy. I fill a basin with hot water from the stainless-steel container on the woodstove. I take a clean washcloth to our back bedroom, so at least I put in effort.

I don't do well by myself. As soon as I have to stop looking strong and positive in front of our family, I crumble from the strength it takes to carry such pretense. I sit down on the bed and stare at the spot where Madi once slept in peace. One of her baby blankets lies tucked in the corner of our bed. Unable to help myself, I reach over and pick it up. Desperate to feel her presence, I lift the blanket to my nose and surround myself with her sweet baby essence. The emptiness brings up images of love chased by despairing pain. Being alone on the tundra. Calling out. Begging for help. Doing CPR on her lifeless body. Hearing her last screams, knowing all she wants is the comfort of my arms and love. Instead, I take her on a ride, ignoring her cries. Blood. Numb. Hollow. Soul-ripping pain. All at the same time.

As if Dave can sense my anguish, he comes into our bedroom and takes the blanket from my tight fingers. Holding it up to his own nose, he closes his eyes. As he opens them, they are raw, hurt, and empty. Rather than hiding his eyes, he looks into mine. Without talking we understand that we can just be with each other in acknowledgment of equal suffering.

Lost in a labyrinth of grief, we will find our way out, together. Yes, we are getting married. Hope triggers direction—forward direction.

"Time to get ready," I say.

He nods his head but takes time to lean over, holding on. This time, he needs my strength. I find that I have it. For him I have it. I hug him in reassurance that we will make it.

Moments go by, and Dave's breathing stabilizes. "We got this," he says.

We each put on our cleanest pair of Carhartt pants. His are black and mine are brown. I find a black tank top that is clean, and Dave puts on a black long-sleeve shirt.

"I have something for you," he says.

I raise my eyebrows.

He brings out a box from a nearby shelf and hands it to me. "Until we can get our rings tattooed on, I thought you might want this."

Mystified, I open the box to see a small ivory figurine on a chain necklace.

"It is a Billiken. For good luck. I got it in Shishmaref and was waiting for the right time to give it to you. We need good fortune, now more than ever."

I agree and put it around my neck. I walk out to show Mom and Dewey.

Dewey jumps up and proclaims, "Rub his tummy, tickle his toes, good luck follows wherever he goes. As a blues chaser, he's a honey, for good luck, just rub his tummy." Dewey laughs with a sparkle in his eye. "It's the Billiken charm. You know, in Japan they are the 'God of Things as They Ought to Be.'"

No surprise Dewey knows that. As a lifelong teacher, spending over a decade in rural Alaska schools, he has picked up a few things. Dave and I find that our families have been creative in our absence. Mom gifts Dave with a bowtie made from camo-green mosquito netting and duct tape.

"It's perfect!" I exclaim.

"Just you wait," Mom says.

Cindy runs over. "Close your eyes."

I play along as she puts a bridal veil over my head. I open my eyes and cry when I see what they made. The veil is an elastic mosquito net and

Mom has somehow sewn on a long matching piece from a mosquito-net tent. A bow connects the pieces of material together with a piece of blue lace woven in.

Mom catches my eye and says, "Something blue."

My warm tears express gratitude. "I can't believe you guys have come up with this. It is so amazing. Thank you so much," I rush on. "I mean it. Thank you so much for making this day as beautiful as possible."

Camp teacher Eric can't resist the opportunity. "You ain't seen nothing yet. Wait until you hear the ceremony. Nothing but pure, divine eloquence and the grace of doves."

The ceremony takes place behind our house up on the hill, overlooking Kobuk Lake. The springtime sun shines off the snow and ice, requiring all of us to wear our darkest sunglasses. Over my Carhartt pants, I wear a deep-green velvet parka with a black wolverine ruff. This was a gift from Dave earlier in the year. Sandra brought out flowers from Alaska Commercial grocery store in Kotzebue. Dave and Alan each put on a daisy—bright yellow, my favorite color. Sandra gives my mom and sister pink carnations to carry. As we walk outside, Dave and I grip each other's hands. We don't let go (see fig. 26).

The ceremony goes by in a blur as Eric, now nervous, starts the proceedings. Our interlocked hands grip even tighter when we say, "I do."

"You may now kiss your bride," Eric says.

People around us all cheer.

Dave lets go of my hand to remove the veil from my face. He leans in to kiss me, and I hear Alan say "Oh man …" as Dewey says "Shh." Dave and I laugh as the world goes back to normal, locked in each other's arms.

The clapping and hollering interrupt us, and we grab hands again. We turn to our family.

Cindy runs up to Dave in a big hug. "Hey, big brother!"

Still holding Dave's hand, I look at my mom and just laugh. It overjoys Mom and me at how Cindy adores Dave. Dave took Cindy under his wing and will do anything for her. As we take pictures, Alan pretends he is falling asleep. Such a kid (see fig. 27).

After the ceremony, our camp neighbors Aggie and Diane host a potluck. Friends come from Kotzebue, bringing an amazing assortment of foods to share. The wedding cake has three tiers. When it's time to cut it, I can't resist the opportunity to smear frosting on Dave's face. He gets me back by kissing my neck with his frosting-covered lips. Friends bellow in amusement. We dance through the evening as our host, Aggie, plays the fiddle. Dave and I make our escape, grateful for how our friends and family came together to find a sliver of joy in each other's company. It is our wedding night. Dave and I hold each other tight, holding back grief and despair so it can't ever rip us apart.

▸FUTILITY

KOBUK LAKE, ALASKA | 2002

As a candle cannot burn without fire,
so man cannot live without spiritual force.

—RAMAKRISHNA

Family and friends leave over the next few days. The shock wears off, and I cross into a state of bottomless despair. People come and go from camp, which requires that I keep things together and try to appear strong. I smile at the appropriate times and engage in mandatory conversations going on around me. Friends bring food and news from around town to let us know they care. They can't change things, but they understand loss and tragedy.

I struggle to sit and listen to small talk. Chuck Schaeffer and Aggie Nelson come over to check on things at the house. Dave went to town with Alan for a couple of days, and I stay home to feed the animals. I make coffee and put out some baked bread to snack on. I can't understand what they are saying anymore, and the small cabin walls cave in on me. I can't breathe. I go outside to cold springtime air. I have to run. I have to find her. My womb spasms with pain, like I am being ripped in half. I can't think of anything except our baby girl. Without winter gear, I stumble through the snow for a quarter of a mile to her grave site. I lie on the frozen ground beneath her wooden cross, wishing I could sink into the dirt and be with her again. My head scrambles, torturing me with shame and guilt, hoping to capture some significant item to cling on to. My thoughts turn to past unhealthy coping skills. Cutting into my skin might bring temporary emotional relief but won't bring her back. My blood dripping on the snow will only remind me of her blood dripping out of her nose.

After an hour, Chuck and Aggie accept that I am a rude host today. Chuck worries about my abrupt departure and searches for me. He finds me and picks me up off Madi's tundra grave, freezing, and brings me inside.

"You need to find something to latch onto in life. No matter what it is," he says. "It might be temporary until you find a more sustainable reason to live. Find something."

I look out the windows to see the spring giving birth to new life all around us. I wish Madi could witness this. Trusting that Chuck knows something about this, I pick something. It can't be me, so I choose Dave.

Months pass by—months of sleepless nights and listless days. I pretend to be strong for Dave, who is my only hope. In Dave there is strength I can cling to. I experience happiness with Dave. Our love pulls me out of deep water, but I still struggle to keep my head above it. I want to become pregnant again. Each month, my period plunges me into a cycle of deep grief. I fixate on things that need work, but inside I am dead and inconsolable. One day, after we take a trip into Kotzebue, I ride on the back of our four-wheeler up to camp.

I scream inside my head as loud as I can, "Help! Help me! Whatever god, spirit, or spirits are out there hanging out by me I need *help!*" I have made similar desperate pleas only a few times in my life. Such desperation often occurs before things turn around. I am ready.

▸HOPE

KOBUK LAKE, ALASKA | 2002

To laugh is to risk appearing the fool.

To weep is to risk appearing sentimental.

To reach for another is to risk involvement.

To expose your feelings is to risk exposing your true self.

To place your ideas, your dreams, before a crowd is to risk their ridicule.

To love is to risk not being loved in return.

To live is to risk dying.

To hope is to risk despair.

To try is to risk failure.

But risk we must, because the greatest hazard in life is to risk nothing.

People who risk nothing, do nothing, have nothing, are nothing.

They may avoid suffering and sorrow;

But they cannot learn, feel, change, grow, love, or live.

Chained by their attitudes they are slaves;

They have forfeited their freedom.

Only a person who risks is free.

—JOURNAL ENTRY, AUGUST 12, 1994

Four months after Madi died, I gratefully learn I am pregnant. The suffering lessens slightly, and I can look toward the horizon now. This time will be different. I have lost my ignorant optimism. Shit happens. Life doesn't always go on. Damned if I test fate with blinders on again. Some things are just beyond our control. Whether it be a random roulette wheel or a master plan larger than we can conceive of. We cannot control everything; we just need to do the best we can.

Instincts tell me our baby is another girl, and I know what I want her name to be. I have to creative about how I present her name to Dave and Alan so I am not overruled. I create a homework assignment for Alan on early women aviators and, surprise, Alan selects to write a report on Amelia Earhart.

"Wow, Alan. Wouldn't that make a great name for your sister, assuming the baby is a girl?" I ask.

"Yeah, that would be awesome. She'll be famous. All the Amelias I know, Amelia Bedelia and Amelia Earhart, are famous."

I agree.

"Amelia is a strong name for a strong gal," Dave chimes in, listening to our conversation.

Amelia Keith it is.

We move into the new house and work hard to finish it before our new baby arrives. She is a great incentive. I listen when Dave suggests I sit down, take a break, or drink water. We live in a white wall tent inside the log-frame house. My sister, Cassie, comes up for the summer to learn about Alaska, and she has to rough it. No running water, gas lanterns, and cold nights. Cassie is fourteen-years-old and a total pleasure to have around. Fun-loving and eager, my sister and I have a lot in common. Cassie learns how to drive the four-wheeler, shoot a gun, chop wood, and other useful Alaska skills. Having my sister by my side keeps the summer positive as we build new memories together. After being away from each other for a few years, it is wonderful to build up a connection with her again.

Our house has a cluttered, lived-in feel while we build around us. Dave builds me a desk using some lumber he milled and stained with linseed oil. I have our camp phone on it, along with an oil lantern for late-night work when the generator is off. My Federal Firearms License paperwork has a home on the makeshift shelves. Alan can sit by me on an old couch, with his camouflage mosquito-net jacket, and do his homework. We have a big white tarp hanging down from the ceiling to serve as a shower curtain. A black water trough serves as the basin, and Dave rigs up a bucket with a spout on it for the hot water we heat on the stove. Dave wires a battery-charging station so that when the generator is on, we can charge the twelve-volt batteries. When the generator is off, these batteries will run our fan and our VHF and AM/FM radios.

Freeze-up comes and goes. I mark the weeks of the pregnancy by keeping close tabs on my "Pregnancy Week by Week" book. November, December, and January creep along. The darkness permeates our lives and dictates our activities. I bake like crazy—nothing wrong with baking when you're pregnant—and have a sale every couple of weeks, trying to save up money. When not busy on the house or baking, our ever-growing zoo also keeps me preoccupied. We now have two Icelandic horses named Hesta and Alvon, a milking goat named Buttercup, two turkeys, five ducks, twenty-five chickens, seven dogs, and one cat (see fig. 28).

I have a fascination with the Arctic sky, whose drastic mood swings match my own—one hour dark and glum, the next full of angelic rays, clouds, stars—the palette of colors more poetic and sublime than the passes of the Sierra Nevada. I will teach our baby all about the sky. Many things come and go in life. The sky reminds us there are great works in the making. We only need to stop, watch, and wonder. We can create miracles. If our girl can look up and know she is a part of something bigger than herself and feel connected, we will accomplish our job as parents.

As my due date draws near, I swing between pessimism and optimism, dread and hope, excitement and terror. I visit my family in Minneapolis for the last two months of pregnancy. On the one-year anniversary of Madi's death, I am eight months pregnant and shopping for newborn clothes. I skip themes that Madi wore such as Winnie-the-Pooh and the one-year-old clothes she should be wearing.

Dave and Alan join me in Minnesota, where Amelia arrives two weeks early. In my vulnerability, the delivery at Regions Hospital scares me. I cannot protect her. I swear I will recognize the preciousness of life and its fragility.

Amelia arrives on March 22, 2003. The minute I see Amelia, her gorgeous innocence erases any outstanding fears. I stare at her face as she thoughtfully takes in the world around her. Her bright-red hair bespeaks her soul's intention to make its unique mark on this world. A twinkle in her eye hints at a sense of humor and wit, while her intense gaze indicates her great compassion and empathy. Tiny soft hands reach up to touch my cheek, and my heart melts. She is mine and I am hers. Dave and Alan each take their turn getting to know precious baby Amelia. For once, Alan is stunned into silence and doesn't make a single joke. Who knows what those two are communicating about? He is probably psychically uploading Archie comic books to her brain.

In April, after Amelia is a few weeks old, we begin the trip back to Alaska. Once in Kotzebue, we need to take Amelia back home on a snow machine under my parka. She is now the same age as Madi. Dave drives, and Amelia and I are in a sled, where I can watch her every second. Once home, the woodstove heat radiates, thawing the frozen, still-uncompleted log cabin.

The next six months go by in blissful harmony, and we fall into a routine as a whole family—at least the four of us (see figs. 29 and 30).

►FOOTPRINTS

CAPE ESPENBERG, ALASKA | 2003

The purple daisy
Soaking in the morning's sun
Welcomes my spirit.

JOURNAL ENTRY, AUGUST 2, 1999

That summer, Dave, Alan, Amelia, and I take a two-week boat trip to look for mammoth ivory along the bluffs and rivers between Kotzebue and Shishmaref. Dave's parents taught at the Shishmaref school for many years, so Dave is familiar with the land and people (see fig. 31).

Shishmaref is a long way by boat—ninety miles southwest of Kotzebue—but we take the scenic route. We gather abundant supplies as we travel with our boisterous six-month-old. In Kotzebue, we stop at Alaska Commercial for groceries and Crowley for two drums of gasoline and oil for the outboard.

We pass through the channel to get around the shallow waters and sandbars and head southeast, following the bluffs of the Baldwin Peninsula, where Kotzebue residents travel with four-wheelers to hunt for finds. The oversearched bluffs hold little interest for us in our quest for mammoth ivory, but this is a great place to walk along the beach. The bluffs, sixty feet tall, generate a rich organic-compost smell from thawing permafrost. Mammoth ivory has a color like permafrost mud and is shaped like a tree root. We examine the bluff base, beach, and shallows for fallen tusks. Dave's more experienced eye discredits my visual findings.

Getting back in the boat, we continue southeast towards Chamisso Island and Eschscholtz Bay. Chamisso is a hidden treasure of northwest Alaska. A tiny natural reserve, two miles long and less than a quarter mile wide, this island, along with the nearby Puffin Island, are home to thousands of nesting birds, including kittiwakes, murres, and of course, puffins. This birder's paradise swarms with birds during certain times of year. As we go around the island, the sandy bird haven stuns me. Marine mammals abound. Three porpoises follow alongside and play with our boat for five miles. These waters are also known to have orca and belugas. There are tents set up on the beach—people enjoying the designated wilderness area. We decide not to stop because our destination lies inside Eschscholtz Bay, along the beaches across from Elephant Point.

Eschscholtz Bay itself is shallow, and we cannot get closer than half a mile from the beach. During July this bay is a traditional beluga hunting ground for the people of Buckland, Deering, and nearby villages. Back in the last ice age, Elephant Point was a herding ground for the mastodons. Only a hundred years ago, it was a reindeer herding ground. Material washes away from Elephant Point and ends up on the northern side of the bay. We anchor the boat out in calm water. Walking half a mile to the beach doesn't pose too big a challenge, except that I need to wear clunky hip waders and carry Amelia on my back in knee-deep water.

Arctic summers can be cold, so I grab sufficiently warm gear and jump over the boat into knee-deep water. I put on my leather shoulder holster with my titanium .38 Special +P. This lightweight revolver affords a level of protection in case any unexpected guests visit. I put a light metal-frame baby carrier on my back, and Dave leans over to put a happy, somewhat sleepy, Amelia in her carrier. I test out the ocean bottom to determine how mucky it will be. Dave and Alan join me with their rucksacks on. Dave is in charge of the rifle because this is an area known for bears. Alan is in charge of snacks. We take about thirty minutes to slog our way in. The wide beaches have dark sand. I walk with my head down and Amelia in tow, beachcombing my way to the east. Dave and Alan do the same, although Alan seems more interested in skipping rocks. I plan to search for hours. A pervasive sense of ancient history overwhelms me as I notice all the fossilized bones and mineralized ivory chips that have broken down over thousands of years. Some bones are from miniature horses and saber-toothed cats. A friend of ours found a saber-toothed cat skull close to our current location. Lost in imagination, I wander (see fig. 32).

Amelia works up an appetite and breaks me out of my reverie. I stop to nurse her. I lay down a blanket for her to roll around on the beach. Together we scour the area surrounding the blanket. Amelia eats a few fossils. We find an object pointing up out of the sand about four inches. Amelia and I dig it out and pry it free. We wash it with seawater and discover a fossilized walrus tusk—our first find. We keep searching and discover a plethora of cool mammoth-ivory pieces. Dave finds a massive mammoth tooth. These are beautiful pieces, even intact, but local carvers make incredible jewelry with them. The color patterns are fascinating.

We need to travel before the calm weather disappears. We eat a lunch of sandwiches, nuts, cheese, and water. A portable cook stove heats water for a hot cup of French press coffee with beans from D&M Coffee in Ellensburg, Washington.

We set off again in search of a protected harbor for the boat. With twenty-four hours of daylight, it's easy to push ourselves into the very early hours of the morning. Our destination is a shelter cabin at the mouth of the Kiwalik River. Stopping once along the way to pick up driftwood for a fire, we park the boat for the night and get out to explore an old dredge parked here long ago during the gold rush, when Candle was a thriving town of twenty thousand people.

The community of Kiwalik used to support mining operations in Candle. They have since abandoned it, and time has broken the old buildings down, giving it a strong ghost town vibe. Nine miles up the river is the old mining town of Candle, which has several current dwellings and a runway. In 1908 Candle served as a turnaround for the All Alaska Sweepstakes, the first major dog mushing competition.

We stay at the shelter cabin for the night. Dave makes a fire inside the shelter cabin and brings in our gear. With Amelia's help, I cook up dinner.

Alan entertains himself by exploring the area. Exhausted, we fall asleep. Early that morning, nature calls. I walk outside to find that the vastness and stillness strikes a chord of peace. For breakfast, we make hot water for the oatmeal before continuing west twenty-five miles to the village of Deering.

Deering is a coastal community on the mouth of the Inmachuk River, with a population of around 130 people. Nearby Cape Deceit, two miles out of town, provides a stunning backdrop for the village and serves as a nesting area for thousands of birds.

We continue toward Shishmaref. We stop to admire the bluffs and stunning rookery of Cape Deceit. Puffins and murres circle us everywhere. After some birding with binoculars, we take the boat forty miles northwest to Cape Espenberg. Cape Espenberg boasts of being one of the earliest Iñupiat settlements in western Alaska. Expecting a three-hour boat ride, we hope to get across Kotzebue Sound before the water gets rough. Southeast winds pick up late in the day. An hour into our ride, swells are large and the sea gets choppy.

"Baby, can you please take the wheel?" Dave asks, calm as ever. "I'd like to secure our gear."

My body comes alive and alert in the rough water.

Alan peaks his head out of the front of the boat, where he was napping. "How is she sleeping?"

I look at Amelia tucked and wrapped up like a burrito in her converted boat seat. To my shock, she has fallen asleep in the now jarring ride (see fig. 33).

"What a kid," we say in unison.

Dave takes ownership of the wheel after covering everything with tarps and checking the boat's battery connection, water filter, and gas tank. I serve as the navigator and stand guard over sleeping Amelia while Dave drives, keeping us pointed in the right direction and changing our angle of attack on the waves as the water current pushes us off track.

The rough seas continue for another couple of hours, increasing in intensity, when we smell gas. The bouncing has cracked our plastic drum gas tank. Gas leaks out over the deck at an alarming rate.

Dave yells, not in panic, but so I can hear him over the waves, "Kat, grab the wheel. Alan, stand by Amelia."

We go to our posts. I keep the deck as level as possible for him. Water splashing against the windshield makes seeing a challenge. The swells—close to ten feet—rise over the top of our tiny fiberglass boat.

Dave works to avert catastrophe and minimize the loss of gas. Could it explode if a spark lands on the gas? Rather than letting my imagination get the better of me, I focus on driving. Dave tips the drum of gas on its side to stop the biggest leak. We have space in another drum to pump gas into. Dave grabs a hand pump and transfers thirty gallons of fuel from the leaking drum into other containers. He jury-rigs another fuel hose intake for the second drum. I flip the switch to start the bilge pump to clear gas out of the boat. Incoming water from the waves rinses the gas away as the bilge works hard to keep up. Drill in hand, Dave fastens the new drum to the boat with a snow machine belt. He wants no similar complications. Twenty minutes after the leak, everything is in order.

Coming back into the cabin to catch his breath, we do some mental math on our options.

Dave sighs. "It's eighty miles to continue to Shishmaref and thirty miles to go back to Deering."

"How much gas do you think we have left?" I ask,

"We need at least forty gallons of gas to get to Shishmaref. If the water stays rough, maybe more. We lost over twenty gallons, leaving us with fifty. We can continue as long as we wait for smooth water from Cape Espenberg to Shish."

"Fine by me!" Alan says.

Amelia, now awake and hungry, states her opinion. She doesn't care where we go as long as she gets to eat. Nursing her in the tumultuous conditions is difficult. Alan unbuckles Amelia and holds her on the floor of the boat. I squeeze into the front crawl space of the cabin.

Dave laughs. "I'll keep her under fifty miles per hour."

Not sure I appreciate his joking at the moment, I laugh anyway. The nonsensical laughter in the frightening and overwhelming conditions removes the tension from my shoulders. Feeling safe with Dave at the wheel, I take Amelia and remove enough of my soaking-wet outer gear to access my soaking-wet inner gear. Breastfeeding is not for sissies. I brace my back in one corner and press my feet against the wall and a toolbox to stabilize our position in the steep undulations. This is when I discover that I get seasick in close spaces.

Time passes interminably before we pull into the calm waters of the shallow, protected lagoon of Cape Espenberg. The boat sighs in relief. Sitting in stunned silence, a comatose daze, we take in our surroundings. Disembarking, we walk up to the cabin to find Johnny Weyiouanna and his relatives from Shishmaref. They greet us with open arms. Right away, Johnny grabs Amelia and sits down with her on the grass. It is a great welcoming committee. They bring us to a hot woodstove to dry off and offer us percolated coffee, caribou soup, and pilot bread crackers. We are royalty at this point. Genuine hospitality is a priceless gift.

My bruised body relaxes in the dry heat radiating from the woodstove. I stare out the window and take in the landscape. Tall, green grass covers the terrain. Not at all worried about the southeast wind assault, but dancing and laughing as if playing a secret game with mother nature. This beach is unusual for the area, with fine-grained sand sculpted in a Zen-like array of ripples left from the last high water. Ripples of memory stay etched in the sand as if to say, "I was here."

Snippets of surrounding conversation pass through my meandering mind.

"Caribou upriver last night," says Perry, one of Dave's longtime friends.

"Still there, you think?" Dave says.

Perry shrugs. "Might as well find out."

"How long can you folks stay for?" Ardith asks. Ardith is Johnny's wife and the matriarch of the family.

Dave puts his feet on a stump closer to the woodstove to better dry out his wet socks. "We're your guests and don't want to impose."

Expecting the incoming hit, Dave flinches as Perry slugs him in the shoulder. "Come on, brother Dave! Don't be stupid!"

"Ow! If I had boots on, I'd chase you."

Ardith finds Amelia and snuggles up with her in a chair by the woodstove. "That isn't an issue," she says. "We hope you'll stay for a few days. Get caribou."

I smile and take another sip of the delicious coffee.

Dave and others hop on Perry's boat and head up the Goodhope River. I take Amelia to our boat to reorganize and clean it after the chaotic trip. Things need to dry out. Dave, Perry, and the guys come back a couple hours later with two caribou. Dave finds three glass fishing buoys, a common discovery along beaches and rivers of the Chukchi Sea. Exhausted, Dave, Amelia, and I crawl back into our boat to sleep. Alan finds a marvelous warm spot to sleep by the woodstove.

The next morning, we wake up to the delicious smell of sourdough hotcakes and fresh caribou meat frying on the woodstove. I am eager to walk the beaches and eat my fill to keep my energy up. I don my revolver holster before settling Amelia in her carrier, hoisting the ensemble on my knee, and whirling her around onto my back. Alan stays and plays with the other kids. Dave helps Johnny with a construction project.

Amelia and I plan to walk the weather-beaten shoreline for hours. The beach is a hundred yards wide at the narrowest point and stretches for miles. Each wave that crashes ashore brings the possibility of seeing ancient wonder. Glass floats, bones, ivory, artifacts, carvings— everything that a hobby archaeologist at heart, like myself, dreams of and more.

Stopping to feed Amelia, I see remnants of sod houses from a thousand years ago. These people lived a very difficult but rich life. They woke up every morning on this beautiful beach with berries on the grassy tundra, fish to catch, and caribou to hunt. I wonder if they accepted the age-old truth: while tough, life punctuates suffering with simple, profound moments.

The hike resumes until I come across a large set of fresh bear tracks. I freeze and scrutinize my surroundings, assuming every dark piece of driftwood in the distance will move and charge us. The *plus* in the +P of my revolver's name doesn't give me much confidence as I visualize being confronted by a charging, hungry bear.

I walk quickly on the way back, feeling like a coward. I force myself to scrutinize objects on the beach, as if to thumb my nose at any bad luck out there trying to thwart my nice day. Vulnerable and alone, I would rather be a coward than miles from Dave and helpless with Amelia. Been there, done that, lost. I run back while singing an uplifting Dixie Chicks song in a fake-happy voice to Amelia on my back. She enjoys the bumpy pace as if this is a new game.

My thumping heart triggers images of Madi and the cost of the last time I was helpless with my daughter. What am I doing out here? How can I bring Amelia out like this, not knowing with surety that this little adventure of ours is 100 percent safe? Panic sets in. Footprints in the sand haunt me, as do the footprints of my past, etched in the landscape of my soul like ripples in the sand. Three more miles to go before we are back to camp. I am alone. Tears mix with sweat and sand. I need to hold Amelia. I pull the carrier off my back, take Amelia out, and sit down in the fine sand. Hugging her, she is the air I need to breathe. Her heart beats against mine. Her little fingers tug my hair.

I spot a figure walking toward us on the beach. I recognize Dave's gait. He came to find me. Safety and security wash over me with immediate effect. Amelia is not in danger. Dave has snacks and sits down by us on the beach.

He sees my tears and needs not ask what is wrong. "It's okay, baby," he says.

Amelia yells out a few happy baby sounds and throws herself in her daddy's arms. He tosses her up and down a few times, and she rewards us with a symphony of giggles. Amelia's carefree laughter drives away the fear-induced black pit that formed a suffocating knot in my throat and stomach. Tears escape my eyes again—tears of relief, love, and new life, tears of appreciation for the gentle strength of my husband and the gift of life that Amelia brings to all around her (see fig. 34).

The next day, we travel to Shishmaref, where more kind, warmhearted friends and family greet us. Part of the reason for making the trip is to purchase carvings. Some of the best carvers in the state live here. The elegant mastery and showmanship of their work is unprecedented and makes the higher price of their art well worth it. We visit for a couple days, taking time to look at a lot of carvings and bracelets. After gassing up, completing boat repairs, and resupplying, we head back to Kotzebue. Stormy weather is two days out, and we cannot afford to take the scenic route home. After our absence, things need tending to.

▸GOODBYE

KOBUK LAKE, ALASKA | 2003

Who loves the rain

And loves his home,

And looks on life with quiet eyes,

Him will I follow through the storm;

And at his hearth-fire keep me warm;

Nor hell nor heaven shall that soul surprise,

Who loves the rain,

And loves his home,

And looks on life with quiet eyes.

—FRANCES SHAW

Dave and I decide that I should take the kids and spend freeze-up in both Minnesota and Washington visiting family. Amelia, seven-months-old now, is still fragile. We aren't comfortable with her being out at camp without the means to travel to town in an emergency. During freeze-up, we can't travel by boat or snow machine or even airplane because the little gravel spit that sometimes doubles as a runway washed out during the last large storm. Dave must stay to keep an eye on the place during this tumultuous time of year when the ice is forming on Kobuk Lake. His homemade airboat project is near completion, and he plans to test it out this freeze-up.

We catch the 5:00 P.M. flight out of Kotzebue, heading down toward

Seattle. Amelia is oblivious to the packing chaos. Alan, now twelve-years-old, knows the routine from years of traveling with his Dad. To help me pack, Dave keeps Amelia close to him. He cradles her in his high-seated captain's chair which he pulls close to the woodstove. He wears the same old well-worn green KOTZ Radio hat and a maroon sweatshirt that settles on his tall muscular frame. His ceramic coffee mug rests on the corner of the woodstove to maintain its warmth. We will sacrifice many things, but good coffee is not one of them. Wearing fleece pajamas, Amelia squeals in pure happiness as she helps her dad prepare his favorite breakfast: homemade bread toasted on the woodstove. Dave can spend hours with his little girl. He makes a funny face, and Amelia giggles carefree, as only babies can. I glance over every few minutes, enjoying the peace of heart that comes from this joyful scene. After losing Madi, both Dave and I understand how we need to cherish these precious moments. We don't know when they will be our last.

It is October and Kobuk Lake is freezing. The boat ride into Kotzebue will be cold. I pack our cold-weather gear for the ride in. Alan and I carry gear out to the four-wheeler trailer and pull a tarp over it to keep our luggage dry. Low temperatures freeze the ground, but we will be driving along the beach, where water and ice would splatter our bags. Alan starts the four-wheeler up after filling the tank with gas. At ten o'clock, the sun is up, and light reflects off the frozen ocean. Frozen ocean? Dang. We have to drive our boat. How is this going to work? Alan and I walk back into the house to report on the conditions.

"Um, Dave, the lake is covered in ice. How are we going to make it?" I ask.

"It's not that thick. No, it's not. It's not too thick," he replies in a playful high-pitched baby-coddling voice. It is hard for him to be serious with Amelia on his lap beaming up at him with adoring eyes.

Alan and I roll our eyes at the same time. We will get nowhere right now.

B. B. King plays in the background, "There Ain't Nobody Here but Us Chickens." Dave sings to Amelia and dances with her by bouncing her up and down on his knee. He doesn't seem to care all that much if we don't make the trip to Ellensburg. It's obvious he isn't excited for us to be leaving.

Meanwhile, I freak out, unwilling to stay at camp during freeze-up with no way of getting medical help if something happens to Amelia. Too much can go wrong. But I don't want to be without Dave for a month.

I ask him to reconsider. "Please, Dave. Can't you come with us? Your mom and dad want to see you. The cabin will be fine. The boats will be fine. We can work down in Ellensburg. Just come with us."

"I wish I could," he says. "Remember last year? The ice came up so high it almost destroyed Aggie's summer house. I'll pull the boat out of the water at camp. We can't leave it in town. Nowhere safe to put it. I'll just stay at home and work on the airboat. I want us to stay here during break-up next year. We can get a safe ride into town anytime once I have this airboat done. I need to finish it."

The death of Madi affects us both in different ways, but neither of us will be helpless anymore. His airboat design is elegant and lightweight, with a frame built from thin spruce lumber he milled over the summer. Tireless, he pushed himself to finish the airboat, hoping it could be ready for freeze-up, but we are out of time.

I make Alan a cup of hot chocolate and grab a cup of coffee off of the woodstove. We finish listening to B. B. King as we watch the outside world come alive with light. The natural light is bright enough that I can turn off the propane lanterns inside the house. The next song plays on KOTZ, "Who Let the Dogs Out?" This is a family favorite.

Alan jumps up and yells, "Woof, woof, woof! Who let the dogs out?" Alan runs over to grab Amelia from Dave.

She yells out her own version of "Woof, woof, woof." Amelia idolizes her big brother and will do anything he wants her to. Alan lies down on the floor with her straddling his neck. She stretches down to grab a ton of Alan's thick, dark hair before latching onto his nose. Amelia knows it is her inherent duty to torture her big brother. She leans down, bites his nose, and drools all over his face.

"Ah! Gross!" Alan yells out, causing baby Amelia to laugh until she falls off him onto the floor.

Dave runs over to join in the fun, picks up Amelia, and yells out, "Diaper Bomb!" Dave holds her high over his head then "drops" Amelia's butt right on onto Alan's face. "Diaper Bomb!" he yells out again as Alan playfully tickles Amelia, hoping to get her soggy diaper off his head. "Who let the dogs out?" Dave sings.

"Woof, woof, woof," Amelia and Alan both yell, in very different dialects.

Drinking my coffee in the wooden rocking chair, looking out over the water, I laugh at their hysterics. Inside, I remain anxious about the trip ahead. I can't shake this tangible sense of dread and unease that follows me around a lot these days. I continue with preparations until we complete the packing process.

The four-wheeler ride down to the boat is frigid. Water from under broken shore ice splashes on our legs. The offshore ice looks solid enough to not want to drive a boat through it. Dave pulls at the anchor cemented in frozen mud with ropes coated in ice. He doesn't seem fazed. Putting on insulated hip waders, he grabs a tuuk—a metal ice chisel on a long pole—from the trailer, and walks through the ice, breaking his way around the perimeter of the boat. Alan pretends he is a giant squashing icebergs. Five minutes later, they climb up on the slippery edges of the boat to break the ice from around the outboard. On cold nights, Dave keeps the lower unit underwater, so the water lines won't freeze. Once done, he clenches the fuel pump multiple times to prime the engine before turning the ignition key. It starts right up despite my worries of a dead battery.

He comes back to shore to help get Amelia aboard and in her boat seat. Amelia loves going on boat rides and is chattering in an excited language only she knows. Foot by foot, we get the boat turned around, breaking the surrounding ice with the tuuk.

In deeper water the ice breaks away from the pressure of the bow of the boat. We plow along at about ten miles per hour into the endless sheet of ice. The ride into town will be long. In meditative wonder, I watch the glare ice roll from the waves our boat creates without breaking. The most rigid ice by our boat breaks away in brittle defiance, while the more flexible sheets undulate with the pressure created by our passage.

We stop a few times to ensure the water pump isn't freezing and continues to circulate water. Alan mans his station in the enclosed boat cabin. For a kid born on the water who doesn't get seasick, this is heaven. He has an Archie comic book and leftover candy bars from the last town trip. Amelia falls asleep with the gentle rocking of the boat and lullaby of the steady scraping of ice. My ears hear the boat complaining as the thin ice scours the fiberglass. I try not to worry. Dave has it under control. He lives by a motto, sometimes irritating, of Safety First. All of us need to have life preservers nearby, ear protection for the four-wheeler and snow machine noise, a survival kit when traveling away from our house, and a back-up plan for the back-up plan. Looking over at Dave, I feel safe and at home. This echoes my impression of him when we first met—him dressed as a mummy and me smelling like dogs and fish. I found a home. Now we are leaving Dave at camp alone. I will be homesick without him by my side. We haven't even left yet, and I ache from emptiness.

Dave and I talk about dreams to come, things we want to accomplish, the businesses we want to develop—small details that maintain our lifestyle. We need a computer to leverage new trends in internet sales. I will negotiate a better wholesale coffee rate from D&M for resale. Alan needs better homeschool books to engage him in the material. Amelia has outgrown her baby clothes and is ready to upgrade to one-year-old sizes. Dave has parts for me to pick up. Small things which paint a dreamy future together we can work hard for.

Two miles from town, the ice becomes thick and takes a long time to break through. Over two hours after we left camp, we arrive and warm up our Dodge truck. Dave drives us to check in at the Kotzebue airport, a small terminal by any standards. There is not much time to spare. We hand our tickets to the boarding agent. I reach up to embrace Dave and realize I am crying. I don't want to be apart. His gentle strength and love make me a better person.

Amelia, Alan, and I line up on the other side of a glass wall that now divides us. Alan, oblivious to sad feelings, is excited for the adventure of a trip. The many new faces distract Amelia. I stare through the glass at Dave who stares back until, after one last, lingering glance, we move away, blocked from his view.

"Goodbye, I will miss you," I whisper to Dave, knowing he can't hear me. My heartache grows with every step away from him.

▸LOST

KOBUK LAKE, ALASKA | 2003

Empty, crow, black sky
gives birth to silence and pain.
No words can bring light.

—JOURNAL ENTRY, JUNE 20, 2019

Freeze-up is underway. During this time of the year, ice forms in large sheets but hasn't solidified enough to travel. During a windstorm, ice can still incur significant damage to property along the beach. Our neighbors, Aggie and Diane, also spend freeze-up out at camp. Dave will help whenever anyone needs it. No matter how big or small the favor, he is someone to count on.

From Ellensburg, I talk to Dave on the phone as much as possible.

"How is the airboat coming along," I ask.

"It is ready for a test run. John Ray is in town and can weld the squirrel cage. I'll take it up the beach later today."

"That is so great!" I say. "How is the plastic working?" Black UHMW plastic covers thin-milled spruce lumber so that the boat can come on and off the ice into the water with little friction.

"Like a charm," Dave says.

"I can't wait to hear how it goes." Dragging the airboat to the beach by himself is a monumental undertaking.

We talk a few hours later that night. "How did the test run go? I ask. "It has worried me all day."

"Don't worry about me. It works great. I tinkered to find the right balance. It is ready to go to town."

I am floored at his progress. "When are you going to go?"

"Not for a while. I'll wait for it to freeze-up better and calm down. It's too windy right now. I don't have the squirrel cage, and there is no need to risk it."

The next morning I have an eye appointment in Ellensburg. These opportunities don't come up often in Kotzebue. Before leaving, I call to say good morning. No answer. I call again. I hang up after the fifth time.

"That's odd," I mention to Dewey.

He reassures me. "Party lines must be busy!" Dewey is familiar with the unreliability of our camp phones.

I go the eye exam but can't shake my sense of unease. The optometrist asks endless questions about our lives. With high energy, as if intoxicated, I answer her questions about Dave and the life awaiting us at camp. We plan to go to Yakima with Dewey to get supplies. I call Dave again from the optometrist's office and still can't get an answer.

"Those darn sunspots are acting up again," Dewey says.

Dewey, Alan, Amelia, and I go on to Costco to get a computer. Dave and I are developing a website to help local artists sell their work. I tell Dewey about our plans, eager to distract myself from this growing knot in the pit of my belly. Alan entertains Amelia in the back seat of Dewey's truck. Before leaving Yakima, we stop for a bite to eat at a local burger joint. I find a pay phone and call five more times. No answer.

Dewey notices my distress. "Can you imagine how often we felt this way? Every day since David moved up there. Those darn phones just never work. Then the next day, David calls us and says he was outside working on logs. Nothing to worry about. Don't you worry."

I appreciate his calm manner. As soon as we get back to Ellensburg, I call Dave and get nothing. I know something is wrong. Dread and fright wash over me.

Preparing for dinner, we get the phone call.

Archie Ferguson (Aggie's son-in-law and our good friend) says, "Hi Kat. Now, don't get upset, but I need to update you."

My breathing stops in knowing. "Go on," I choke out.

Archie continues, "Dave and Diane left camp in the airboat about three hours ago and haven't made it to Kotzebue. Diane had a stroke and needs to make it to the emergency room. Dave carried her in the airboat, having no other option. I am up here on the hill in Kotzebue and can't see any sign of them. It is real stormy right now. Southwest winds. Water is rough with whitecaps and ice."

I am silent and waiting.

Archie asks, "Have you heard from him?"

I say, "I haven't. Are the search-and-rescue crews out? Dave did a test run with the airboat yesterday, but it is too lightweight for bad weather."

Archie says, "Search and rescue can't go out yet. The storm is too bad. Airboats go where and when others can't. When they have problems, others can't help."

Refusing to think we are helpless, I ask, "What about planes? Can they do a flyover?"

Archie says, "Right now the visibility is too low. Eric Sieh will take off when it clears."

At that, I feel a sense of relief. Eric is one of the best bush pilots I know. If anyone knows where to look and can handle the weather, it's him.

"Can I do anything?" I ask.

"No," Archie replies. "If you hear anything let me know. I will do the same. I'm sure they're just stuck on the beach somewhere or the motor broke down. We will find them and bring them home." Archie's voice contains hope but also the pain of wisdom, having supported many unsuccessful searches. Archie and his wife, Lena, volunteer much of their time trying to keep residents of the region safe.

"Thanks," I say and hang up the phone.

Turning around I find a room full of people looking at me with white, drawn faces. This is the day his family has lived in fear of—the day their son is the object of a search. I pack and plan to go home. Alan will stay longer with his grandparents so he doesn't have to live through the fear and stress of a search. He will come home when they find his Dad. The only calls I receive from Archie are those with no news (see fig. 35).

Later that night, Archie calls to tell me that the search is on and official. November 7, 2003. "We still can't do much because of the weather. Eric can't take off. Boats can't go out because of ice conditions leaving the lagoon and in front of town. The only piece of equipment that can make it to where Dave and Diane likely are is Danny Shield's airboat."

"Have you spoken to Danny?" I ask.

"We've been calling all afternoon and got through on the VHF. Their camp phone is down. When Danny heard what happened, he took off right away to look for them, despite the awful weather and the fact it's dark out."

I become worried for Danny now. "Have you heard from Danny? Is he safe?"

"He called on the VHF, but he found nothing. He had to turn around about half an hour ago. He'll try again when it calms down or at least gets light out."

My stomach turns over at knowing, no matter what, there is no help to come for Dave and Diane tonight. Diane, with a stroke, stuck out all night in the nasty, wet, cold, windy weather. I know Dave will do his best to take care of her, but how will she survive?

Amelia and I make it to Kotzebue the next morning. As the fog lifts, airplanes search but boats still can't make it out. The airplanes find nothing—not a single trace of Dave, Diane, or the airboat. On the third day, boats make it out to search. They find Diane's body still inside a part of the airboat. The boat drowned and Diane with it.

Diane was a second mom to Dave and often took care of Alan. A mom herself, with numerous grandchildren, her loss devastates the community of Kotzebue. Diane was only sixty-one years old.

Dave is not with the boat. Dave always wears his float suit when boating in rough conditions. I hope his safety training helps him to stay alive and make his way to shore. My mom, Cassie, and Cindy come up to Kotzebue to stay with Amelia and me during the search. Alan is still in Ellensberg with his grandparents.

The search continues for weeks into freeze-up, but the search transitions to recovery despite my insistence that he must be wandering around on the tundra, trying to make his way back to Kotzebue. Once the ice is thick enough to travel on, search-and-rescue crews drill holes in the ice, looking for any sign of him. Nothing. Eric Sieh gives me the great gift of being able to fly around and search myself even after so many others tried to find him. Chuck Schaeffer spends hours taking a four-wheeler around on the ice, looking for traces of him on the sandbars. They are looking for a body. I am looking for my husband, alive and well.

▶THANKSGIVING

KOBUK LAKE, ALASKA | 2003

If I could only fly, if I could only fly

I'd bid this place goodbye to come and be with you.

—MERLE HAGGARD, "IF I COULD ONLY FLY"

It is twenty days since Dave went missing. Twenty-one days since I heard his voice. Forty-three days since I said goodbye through the glass windows of Alaska Airlines. Is it time for me to accept his death?

It is now time for a snow-machine ride home. I haven't been to camp since the airboat accident and don't know what we will find. We have no snow machines in town, all of ours are at camp, so Dickie Moto lets me borrow his. Amelia, eight-months-old, needs me to think straight. How much gas do we need? what type of food? what supplies? What clothes can I find for her to drive home in? What else do we need to bring? My brain isn't working. My heart breaks more with every beat. Amelia will never see her Dad again—this amazing, gentle giant of a man who adores her. Rather, adored her. Past tense. She will never know his smile like he knew hers.

Mom and Cassie go back to Minneapolis, and I now need to keep Cindy and Amelia safe. That weight falls on my shoulders. Being fifteen, Cindy is still in high school but stays through her winter school break. Time away is not good for her. My sister, with the heart of a lion, will go through any inconvenience to help the people she loves.

Alan isn't with us anymore. After losing his Dad, Dave's parents decide that Alan is better off in Washington with them. When Dave and I married, we didn't think about the legal aspects of living our lives together. I didn't adopt Alan; the thought never occurred to me. I miss him deeply, and I can't think of his smiling face without crying. How is it right for Alan to lose his Dad, his home, his baby sister, his stepmom, and his entire life in Alaska all at the same time?

Cindy stays with Amelia inside our temporary housing in Kotzebue. Packing up the snow machine sled, I wrap our boxes up with a tarp, tie the load with whatever rope I find, gas up the machine, check the oil, and go back inside to get dressed. A blizzard rages outside, complete with high winds, low visibility, and plenty of snow.

"Cindy, do you have enough clothes?" I ask.

"I think so," she says. "Still need a face mask."

Looking over at her misfit hodgepodge collection of borrowed gear, I can't help but laugh. Her bunny boots are about three sizes too big and her down pants are close to a foot too long. Digging through a random box, I find a face mask and throw it her way. The weather isn't great, but we are going home for Thanksgiving.

"Looks great," I say.

Cindy feeds Amelia a breakfast of smashed bananas and cheerios, the remnants of which land all over the kitchen floor.

I pick up Amelia. "Wow, baby bubba, you sure know how to leave your mark on the world."

"She got a few cheerios in her mouth and in my hair," Cindy adds.

I have a pile of clothes for Amelia to wear. This will be new for her. As a super-young baby, Amelia went on snow machine rides, but she won't remember. The big process of layering begins with fleece, mukluks, hats, mittens, then outer jackets. Amelia will ride inside my large fur coat.

My hands are shaking with knowing—knowing I need to bring Amelia out to camp on a snow machine. I feel silly, knowing that this resilient eight-month-old child is healthy and that I have no reason to fear. My gut rears up in disagreement, shouting in remembrance. I have all the reason to fear. Cindy shares my concerns. Neither of us are in a hurry to go, but we both seem to grasp the inevitability of fate. Time to go home.

We take off to camp, drive on an unmarked, blown-over snow trail, and make it home without trouble. Along the way, I can't help but search. Where is Dave? Why can't we find him? He has to be out here somewhere. The three of us make our way through the miles outside Kotzebue, feeling alone and lost in the white wall of snow. How different from times past, when going home meant love, joy, happiness, family, and connection. We now go home to obligation and to a stubborn refusal to give up on a shared dream. I want to hope that Dave will come home, and we need to keep things moving for when he does.

We come home to an empty cabin that has the last remnants of him laying out collecting dust. I feel close to Dave again for the first time since we departed at the Kotzebue airport. His clothes, his smell, his music, his hat, his sweater, his coffee mug, his winter boots, him. Despair is not a cozy companion. The cruel fates that set up this sequence of events nail me to a cross of shame and longing.

A notepad lays by the rotary phone with his handwriting transcribing his thoughts. He was looking at airline tickets to meet us in Ellensberg while we were still there. Was he going to surprise us? He made a note about the band Marc Brown and the Blues Crew and where to find their music. His last cup of the infamous D&M coffee lies on the stones of the wood-stove. His favorite hat hangs from a nail in the center log of our house. B. B. King is on the record player he was listening to the evening after I said goodnight on the phone from far away. The airboat scaffolding is outside the house with tools waiting for Dave to put them away. Life at our house hit the pause button, waiting for Dave's return as if holding its breath.

There is wood in the house left behind from Dave's proactive efforts. Cindy searches for kindling while I load up logs. Within five minutes both woodstoves are roaring. Amelia hangs out in her Dad's captain's chair close to the stove with her outside gear still on. She gets mad that she can't move and cries. I sit down in the chair to comfort her and weep. My rapid breathing catches with every breath as I struggle for control, trying to grip my sense of reality as if I can hold it.

I realize this little baby girl provides me with comfort, not the other way around. Taking a few breaths, I gain control before looking to Cindy.

"What a mess, huh?" I try to take a light tone about the bachelor pad of disarray he left behind. "What a guy! Food on the counter, clothes everywhere, dirty dishes …"

Cindy looks around. "Yeah. How did he manage for two weeks without us?" Cindy goes outside to turn the propane tank on, and I find a book of matches for the pilot lights.

"Thanks, Cindy," I say as she comes back in. "Ready for some coffee?"

"That sounds good."

Amelia calms down, and as the temperature in the house rises, we take off a few layers of gear.

"I'd like to get things done outside the house before the snow covers everything. Want to come out or stay in?" I ask.

Cindy looks at Amelia. "I can stay inside with Amelia."

We tag-team, taking trips to the outhouse and watching Amelia before I head out.

"Holler if you need anything," I say. "I will be right outside."

The priority is always wood. Finding the latest wood pile, I spend time splitting wood before carrying a dozen armloads into our storm shed. I cut kindling for faster fire-starting. The main camp tools are still visible, and I put them away. We need a snow machine. I find our fan-cooled 550cc Polaris on a pallet, where Dave put it last spring. Driving it up on the pallet prevents the snow machine track from freezing into the mud or tundra at times just like now. It takes ten minutes to get it going, and everything sounds in working order. I search around for gas cans and find enough gas for a trip to town. I am not sure which drum has straight-up gas and which, if any, have pre-mixed gas. As a mechanic, Dave didn't trust the oil injection system and disabled it. He preferred to add oil directly to the gas at a ratio of one-to-sixteen. Not finding any mixed gas, I search for some oil.

Confusion sets in, "What kind of oil is it now? Two cycle? Synthetic? Four cycle? Motor oil? Why so many oils?" I shriek out to no one in particular.

Time to get the generator started. I placed it by the woodstove for an hour to warm up. It is standard practice for us to bring it inside every night to protect this crucial piece of equipment. This time however, it was outside for six weeks. That Dave, of all people, left it outside shows the emergency Diane was in. The generator is always finicky, and I worry about damage. I carry it outside and fill it with gas, turn on the fuel valve, choke it, cross my fingers, and pull back on the starting cord. Nothing. Five more pulls. Nothing. Ten more pulls. Nothing. I go through all the steps again, checking the on-off switch and the fuel valve, adjusting the choke setting. Nothing.

"Fuck!" I scream out at the top of my lungs, instantly feeling bad that I've worried Cindy.

It's getting dark out, and I know it is dark inside the house. I need a different plan. I bring the generator back in the house.

"Sorry, Cindy didn't mean to yell out there"

She laughs at me.

"How is Amelia doing?" I ask.

"She's great. Happy to have her bouncy chair back."

Amelia is bouncing and singing an unintelligible song. This was Alan and Amelia's favorite game. With a heart so heavy I can't stand, I tell myself that I have to get some lights on. I go outside to turn the propane bottle connected to a series of copper tubes that end in mantle lanterns. Crossing my fingers, I grab a lighter, turn the valve on the lamps, and wait for the mantle to light. It does! Whew. We light three more and see the house brighten with the soft, warm light of propane lamps. I turn on the VHF radio so we can hear local gossip. Nothing happens—again. The twelve-volt battery it connects to is dead.

I slump by the woodstove in defeat.

Today is Thanksgiving.

"What do you want to do for Thanksgiving?" I ask Cindy.

We glance at each other with tears in our eyes. Thanksgiving without Dave will be a tasteless meal. Growing up, our family always went to Chicago, where my mom took us to visit her sister's family. The meals were massive. The cribbage tournaments and ping pong battles always made it a weekend to look forward to. This isn't Chicago.

Cindy just shrugs her shoulders, unable to respond.

I flop down in the chair and watch Amelia for a long while, letting her joy wash over me.

"It is time for a gourmet Turkey Day dinner—or whatever we can find close to it. Are you hungry, Cindy?" I ask again.

Hungry or not, cooking seems like the next logical thing we can accomplish without failing. We look through the stash of food that remains free of the bear, squirrel, and mouse interference. We find an unopened box of Hamburger Helper and a box of pasta primavera salad.

"Score!" Cindy and I yell out at the same time.

After melting snow, boiling water, and slaving away at the stove for all of five minutes, we have Thanksgiving dinner sitting on a couple of chairs huddled close to the woodstove for warmth. I leave the propane oven door open for extra heat. We eat on paper plates because we don't have enough melted snow water for dishes yet.

It isn't much. The three of us sit there, drowning in grief, all trying to put our strong face forward. We look out the window wondering where Dave is, as if he will drive our way any minute. Every snow machine that comes along our beach fills me with hope and follows with despair when it passes us by. A glass of Thanksgiving Wild Turkey sits in Dave's memory on the wooden stool he carved my name into as a welcoming gift when I first arrived on his doorstep. Amelia calls out for more food and laughs as Cindy gives it to her. Looking their way, I realize I have a lot to be thankful for. Thank you for giving me a daughter. Thank you for my family. Thank you for this place. I will try to understand, damn you, I will try.

▸MAN UP

KOBUK LAKE, ALASKA | 2004

Where you used to be, there is a hole in the world,
which I find myself constantly walking around in
the daytime, and falling in at night.

—EDNA ST. VINCENT MILLAY

Despite the overwhelming odds, I commit and cling to our dream of raising Amelia at camp, to give her a solid foundation in the lifestyle that Dave and I worked hard to provide for her. I cling to the shreds of the life we shared. I owe it to Dave, and so I try.

The practicality of living at camp without him overwhelms me. While caring for Amelia, I need to do all the things Dave was a natural at, such as fixing the snow machine, cutting down trees, hauling water, running the boat, tweaking the generator, and repairing the house. I need to learn to be a welder, electrician, plumber, lumberjack, mechanic, survivalist, and more. I hold a basic awareness of these things but never believed I would be the sole operator of everything. Oh yeah, did I mention money?

Months later, search and rescue calls off the search. I still operate with that tiny pinprick of hope that Dave hit his head and forgot his identity. It isn't until the following spring break-up, May 29, 2004, that they spot Dave's body hanging on a pile of ice in front of Kotzebue.

It is time to say goodbye.

We bury him at the corner of our still-unfinished log cabin next to Madi. In July 2004, family comes out to stay for the funeral. Many community members attend. The City of Kotzebue rents us a jackhammer and a three-thousand-kilowatt generator to dig his grave. Dave's body arrives by boat. The casket travels from the beach to the grave site by the four-wheeler. Chuck makes a large wooden cross to match our daughter's tiny one. Madi's cross reads, "Our Littlest Angel," and Dave's reads, "Our Big Angel." The two crosses stand side by side overlooking the vast horizon of Kobuk Lake (see fig. 36).

I remember little of those days. Things go by in a blur. I ping pong from one disaster and broken-down piece of equipment to the next. People check on Amelia and me at camp. Friends install a stove, bring by coffee, drop off a fish, etc. Autcha Kameroff, her brother Frank, and Ruth-Ann take shifts helping me go to the woodlot and watching Amelia. Perry Weyiouanna helps to finish parts of the house and teaches Amelia to walk. My faith in humanity grows. I don't live in an isolated bubble at camp but in a community that cares for one another (see fig. 37).

Autcha Kameroff comes out to help me sort Dave's clothes. Things that no longer have a distinct purpose go in a big pile and are burned to release his spirit. Another close friend, Tracey Schaeffer, lends constant strength and compassion along with practical parenting-at-camp ideas. Dickie Moto accompanies me to the airboat remains on a gravel beach at Lockhart Point. We watch the boat burn as we both say farewell to our friend.

Dammed up grief overwhelms me like flood waters gushing out of a broken levee. I insulate Amelia, now fifteen months old, from the raw bitterness. I keep him in our hearts through stories, but she won't have memories of her amazing father.

Cindy goes home to Minnesota and is back at school. I continue to work on critical chores and repairs while keeping Amelia safe.

One cold, wet day in September, I wake up to find a leak in the roof. After coffee and a brief examination, I need to climb up to make the repairs. Amelia, an exploratory toddler, is still learning how to balance herself. Feeling confident I can contain her baby enthusiasm, I install a childproof gate on the door opening outside. I am wrong. I am up on the roof, when Amelia pushes her body the gate, trying to find me. She succeeds. She makes her way through the doorway and falls over a foot face-first onto an industrial metal grate. The jagged metal surface connects with her nose and rips away the flesh, causing massive bleeding. Hearing her screams, I scramble down from the roof. It looks like she broke her nose. Holding her close, I run to the four-wheeler and drive the mile down to the boat parked in the lagoon.

At the lagoon, I put my screaming baby down. I jump in the water, without waders, pull the anchors, and start the outboard. I strap Amelia into her seat and begin the eighteen-mile boat ride to Kotzebue. Kobuk Lake is rough today, and the jarring bounces cause Amelia pain. Partway to town, I run into Autcha and Ruth-Ann coming back from their camp. Autcha hops into our boat and drives the rest of the way so I can tend to Amelia. Once we park in the boat harbor, we rush across the street to the hospital. They clean up Amelia's wound, strap her down, and give her six stitches down her nose. At least it didn't break (see fig. 38).

January gets cold. We huddle in a bed pushed next to the woodstove because it is forty below and the house lacks insulation. To keep the house warm, I have been keeping two woodstoves going around the clock. To shut the house down for the night, I add wood to the stoves, stock the house with wood so I don't have to go outside at four in the morning, turn off the generator, bring it inside to warm up by the woodstove, turn off the propane lanterns, and blow out the votive candle I often light in memory of Madi and Dave.

Amelia and I are both sick with the flu. We take cold medicine. Being sick, Amelia is restless, crying, and needs Mom to lie down and snuggle with her. Holding her close, I rock her to sleep. Knowing I still need to complete evening chores, I force my eyes open. Hours later, I wake up to find our house filled with smoke and a blazing fire. Our house cat, whose primary goal in life is to keep mice, shrews, and squirrels from getting into our food totes, has knocked over the votive candle and started a fire on the main support log of our house.

I jump up and douse the flames with an extinguisher, but the smoke conditions are extreme. I grab what clothes I can find, wrap Amelia in a massive parka, and go outside. The snow machine is too cold to turn over. I can't start it. Grabbing the generator from inside the smoky house, I start it and point the generator exhaust toward the snow machine carburetors. Amelia coughs. Already sick, her oxygen levels diminish from the smoke. It takes thirty minutes of being outside in the forty below zero temperature before I can start the snow machine and drive us to town.

It is three o'clock in the morning when we arrive in Kotzebue. I can't get the emergency room's attention. I start our unheated pickup and drive around town searching for help. At last, the ER lets us in. Amelia warms up, receives oxygen, and the doctors clear our health to leave.

We have another problem: we have nowhere to go. Camp is a disaster. In a freezing, dark truck, we drive around the lonely town of Kotzebue for hours. Another close call puts Amelia's life in jeopardy. I decide right there, with finality, that it is time to leave camp. In this moment of utter failure, it's time to let go of Dave and the dreams we held together. I know his response to my desperate unasked question. I have to choose the living. There is no choice. We must leave the house we built together. I have to choose Amelia and her life above all. I know what I have to do next, and my heart breaks even further.

Part Four

FINISH LINE

▶ IDITAROD, MILE 446

GALENA, ALASKA | 2015

The deeper that sorrow carves into your being,

the more joy you can contain.

—KAHLIL GIBRAN

A year has gone by since my 2014 rookie Iditarod. I am in the 2015 Iditarod during my twenty-four-hour layover, this time in Galena. I realize subjecting myself to the harsh conditions of this race—the profound fatigue, the vulnerability to nature, the pressure to continue because your life and the lives of your dogs depend on it—leaves me so raw and exposed that I can't help but receive the profound beauty that the wilderness unfurls before me.

If I allow myself to get wrapped up in adversity, the wallowing can wreck my race. If I surrender, ride the waves, some breathtaking gift—a sunset, a moonrise, the northern lights—is always waiting just around a bend in the trail. This is the balance. Not only the race, but life itself.

I leave two dogs in Galena, so I have ten still in the game. After the twenty-four-hour rest is an eighty-two-mile run to Huslia. When I arrive at Huslia, the checkpoint rocks. The community goes way over the top to welcome the Iditarod for the first time. Huslia is an active sled dog community. For miles along the road leading to town, they have signs up encouraging the mushers with positive phrases. The temperatures are sixty to seventy degrees below zero. The northern lights tonight in Huslia will win awards for any ambitious photographer. I stay in Huslia for six hours. The dogs are working hard, and the cold weather is taking a toll on them.

The temperatures from Galena to Huslia to Koyukuk are the lowest I have run dogs in, let alone camped in. When we camp, it is the middle of the night and sixty below. The cooker won't start. It is hard to get Heet to ignite when it's colder than minus thirty-five Fahrenheit. I shiver from cold, so getting the tinder out to start the cooker is a big project. I need to start a fire. Sleeping on the dogsled will not cut it tonight. At such cold temperatures, you need skill to get a roaring fire going. There isn't a ready supply of wood when we pull over to camp. I walk off the trail, break off chunks of dry branches, carry them back through the thigh-deep snow, then repeat. The exertion of finding wood warms my body despite my fingers still freezing. I take care of the dogs, feed them, massage them, and help them lay down before I get my sleeping assembly ready by the small fire. I put down straw, a Therm-a-Rest pad, then my sleeping bag. I invite my lead dog, Ears, to rest with me by the fire.

I am full of discomfort and fear this deep cold. I am accustomed to danger, but one tiny mistake out here could have serious repercussions for me and the team. I calm myself and warm my hands by the fire until I think to look up. Above the black spruce trees that line the trail, I see a dazzling display of northern lights that dance around as if on Broadway. The moon is new, so the stars stand out in bright contrast to the black night sky. They sparkle in harmony with the green, red, and orange fireworks that spread out across the entire expanse of the sky. I won't sleep in the cold temperatures, and this wonder-filled night keeps my rapt attention.

This is the reward for being out. This is my *why*—what I search for. These two hours supply answers to many of my lingering questions. I leave with a better understanding that resisting life's lows is not only futile but foolish—making it impossible to fully experience life's highs. Am I brave enough to allow myself to experience the full range of emotions that life has to offer? A challenge is inherent in this question. The "low" waiting for me, on the horizon, will be a big one given the staggering beauty of the "high" I experienced tonight. These thoughts, and more, occupy my mind as I drift in a waking dream that lures me into times past.

Two days later, I leave Kaltag for Unalakleet with nine dogs. This run tests teams as the eighty-five-mile run can put a lot of pressure on a tired team. Alaska Natives have used this route for thousands of years. It works its way southwest up the Kaltag River valley through a wooded trail. After ten miles, the trail climbs up the south side of the valley to the summit of the portage at eight hundred feet. The difficulty of this section depends on weather and trail conditions such as snow depth, wind speed, and whether there is a trail at all. My few remaining dogs are doing great and maintaining a positive attitude. Nine dogs is still plenty to make it to Nome. I am not concerned. Scratch that. I am a new musher and concerned about every single little detail. How is Loki eating? How are Ear's hips? Do Ripple's shoulders seem sore? Do I have enough spare booties? Where do we rest? Do I take straw? Endless questions come up which keep me concerned that in a sleep-deprived state I might miss some crucial detail that will derail the team and hence the race.

I arrive at the Old Woman shelter cabin, where the Iditarod's more protected inland trail transitions into a stretch along the Bering Sea coastline that leaves mushers and their dog teams exposed to harsh offshore winds. Stories hint that the cabin, named for the nearby Old Woman Mountain, harbors wandering spirits, including the ghost of a woman who died in an avalanche. Iditarod historians warn racers to leave her something, like food, lest bad luck follow them all the way to Nome. Some mushers report hearing the Old Woman humming a haunting melody. I know the legends but remain skeptical. Old Woman is a welcoming place. My plan is to stop for a four-hour rest. I hope for at least one hour of sleep for myself, fortifying me for the last three hundred miles to the finish line.

I stop my team, secure the sled with snow hooks, and get ready to snack the dogs, when I notice blood dripping from the nose of my beautiful, blue-eyed, young leader, Loki. Within two minutes the drip becomes a gush, blood pouring from his nose and mouth—a dark red stain spilling out onto the white snow. Holding him close, I hear a rattling in one of his lungs, and before long he is struggling to breathe. I look around for help, full of worry he has a spontaneous pneumothorax causing blood to pool in his lungs. The Old Woman shelter cabin is not an official checkpoint, and the nearest veterinarians are in Unalakleet, thirty-five miles away.

My leader is in crisis, and my tired team offers our only transportation. I lay out straw so the other dogs don't get stiff. They need rest while I figure out how best to help Loki. Four other mushers are in the shelter. They break their rest to provide aid, each lending their relative expertise and experience to the situation. This is always the case during a crisis for musher or dog. Mushers set aside competition. Averting that crisis and ensuring the safety of all involved becomes the sole focus. It is a fundamental code.

Together, we lay Loki down on what appears to be his stronger side to avoid putting pressure on the weaker lung. We try to get the blood to drain out his mouth rather than going down his throat to the lung. It isn't working, and Loki chokes. Everyone present agrees that Loki will not make it without emergency care. It will take me at least seven hours to get to Unalakleet. My only other option is to push the "help" button on the SPOT Tracker carried by every Iditarod musher. Designed to help race fans watch each musher's progress in the race online, SPOT Tracker technology has advanced to allow for one-way communication. I can send a distress message, calling for a Coast Guard helicopter with one button. With another, I can call for snow machines to rescue us.

The 2015 Iditarod rules dictate that when a musher pushes the help button, they scratch from the race. I have no choice. The more experienced mushers and I all agree. I take the device out of the dog booty pinned on the front of my sled. I lift the cover, and realizing the futility of Loki's situation, I take the irreversible step that ends our race. There is no promise in how long it takes help to arrive.

Lance Mackey, an Iditarod champion with four consecutive wins, drives his team through Old Woman, planning to stop and snack his dogs for a few minutes before moving on. He comes over to see what the trouble is and offers help. Concerned that the snow machines might not get here in time to save Loki, Lance offers to carry my leader in. His dogs travel faster than mine, so I accept. I watch as Lance carries him away, convinced this is the last time I will see Loki alive.

It takes all my strength to refocus on taking care of my remaining eight dogs. Operating on autopilot, I start the dog cooker to melt snow for their dinner. I snack them with frozen sheefish, massage their feet, and go inside the shelter cabin. Gripped as I am by anguish, my attempt to sleep for the remaining hour fails. Once the dogs have their four hours of rest, we set out for Unalakleet to find Loki.

The dogs know something is wrong. I try to hide my distress from them, but after conquering close to seven hundred miles together in seven days, that just isn't possible. Like a tidal wave, all the agony, grief, guilt, and shame from my past swells into an insurmountable tidal wave. It all comes crashing down. Our race is over, Loki will not make it, and it is my fault. In my state of exhaustion, flashbacks come in rapid succession.

I am a destroyer of everything around me with my unquenchable hunger for something more—something that even I don't understand.

It is my fault that my newborn daughter Madi died, this month, thirteen years ago. What right do I have putting precious life in harm's way? My endless hunger for the wilderness seems poor justification. My need for adventure, remoteness, and solitude resulted in their deaths. How can I make others suffer?

The blood dripping from Madi's nose and from the corner of her tiny mouth— the blood dripping from Loki's nose onto the pristine snow—pressing my palms into Madi's fragile chest over and over, praying that the CPR would make her breath again. I scream into the empty air with no help for miles in any direction.

The dogs know a veil between worlds has ripped open. They know I have succumbed to a different reality—one that carries a risk. They slow their pace, unsure of what to do. At moments, I break out of my living nightmare to realize the team has stopped. I run along the sled to get the team moving down the trail again.

The screams of my young daughter Amelia that had sent me flying off the roof, where I was trying to fix a leak—finding her, face covered in blood, nose split open—the jagged tear in her flesh—Amelia screaming in pain. My choice to stay out at camp on my own with my baby daughter after my husband had died in a frozen sea. All my choices cause every living thing around me pain.

It is twenty-five below zero and my whole body shivers. I sink into a dangerous despair, but don't care. This not caring is a feeling familiar from long ago, when I considered myself such a poison that I cut myself.

Blood on the razor blade—crimson drips on the hardwood floor. Memories of abuse forcing their way into my daily life and having flashbacks in the middle of a shopping mall. Nightmares of horror-filled images and never being safe. Lashing out at Josh in bed when all he wants to do is hold me.

I want to fall asleep in the snowbank and not wake up. But my dogs need me to keep going to reach the food and straw that await them in Unalakleet. I must search for the next stake.

I stand on the sled runners as we make our way through the unforgiving landscape. I feel the echoes of pain in my breasts hardened with milk in Madi's absence. Her life is void because of my mistake. Now I've taken Loki's because I missed something—some flip of his ear or change in his gait that should have clued me in to his trouble. I missed something because I'm not good enough. I have no right to be playing with the lives of my faithful companions. Admitting that I am a failure does not even touch the horror caused by my neglectful behavior. The scale on which I inflict hurt on those I love goes far beyond failure and into a realm of living hell. My love is a death sentence.

Seventeen hours after leaving Kaltag, we make it to Unalakleet where I discover that a snow machine met Lance on his way into town and took over carrying Loki in. A team of volunteer race vets took care of Loki and kept him alive. They monitored his lungs and made sure there are no other health problems. Loki is now fine. He inhaled a piece of straw. After hours of running, it caused a vein in his nasal cavity to rupture, which then bled down into his lungs. The outward sign of which was him bleeding from the nose. The fact that Loki survived does little to pull me out of the despair I know is mine to carry.

▸STARTING OVER

ANCHORAGE, ALASKA | 2005

The mark of your ignorance is the depth of your belief in injustice and tragedy. What the caterpillar calls the end of the world, the Master calls the butterfly.

—RICHARD BACH

"Well, Cindy, time to buy a car," I say with a positive voice that doesn't match my grim expression.

"Yay," she says. "What kind do you want?"

Cindy came back to Kotzebue a couple months ago to help pack up camp and move me to Fairbanks. I look around at the Affordable Used Cars lot in Anchorage and say, "I have no clue. What do you think?"

"A truck!"

Happy to have direction, we walk toward a couple of big-looking rigs, when a salesman comes out. Cindy, Amelia, and I walk away hoping to avoid conversation. Big fail.

"What brings you three fine ladies to Anchorage?"

Cindy and I glance at each other trying to not laugh.

"We're looking for a truck we can use in Fairbanks," I say.

"What are you going to do in Fairbanks?"

"I enrolled at the University of Alaska, where I received a financial aid package." Hint, hint—I have little cash. "I am throwing myself into the new challenge of college."

"Good for you!" he says. "College mom. Got it." He backs away inch by inch.

Overwhelmed, I realize that we want his help to get a decent car. "We flew in from Kotzebue this morning, where we live out at a camp," I say. This isn't helping our cause any.

"What will you do?" Cindy whispers, "Trade him a dogsled for a car?"

I suppress a laugh and say, "Maybe a few caribou hides?"

The salesman peers at us, curious and intrigued. "Live at camp by yourself?"—in other words, where is the husband and/or baby daddy?

"Yes, my husband died last year." This is a great conversation killer and works to stop that line of inquiry. "As a single parent, I have to plan for a future that can provide for my kiddo. Time to get a solid education."

"Let me show you around the lot," he says. "Where are you staying? I ask because some Fairbanks cabins are remote and off-road."

"The three of us will live in campus housing to start. It's all about the running water. Plus automatic electric heat." Even saying it feels spoiled, and I already miss camp.

Cindy senses my change in mood and jokes, "I'm sure before long she'll move us all into a log cabin in the middle of nowhere with a woodstove and no running water."

The salesman laughs and says, "I recommend a truck with block heater, oil pan heater, and battery blanket. It's your lucky day. I have just the thing."

We walk with him to look at a large maroon extended-cab diesel GMC truck.

"Oh no," I say at the same time Cindy says, "Oh yes!"

Amelia joins in with, "Yay!" Her vocabulary is still developing.

I am overruled. "Looks good," I say. "How much?"

"Don't you worry about that. I've got ideas to bring the price right on down for you."

Two hours later, after signing my life away, we drive off the lot in what I feel is an oversized yet useful vehicle. I am eager to get on the road to Fairbanks today. It has been a long couple of days preparing to leave camp. The boat ride to town was rough. I found a trailer in Kotzebue to pull the boat up out of the water, but the process was not seamless. At least I won't have to worry about it getting stuck during freeze-up while I am out of town.

A trip to Wal-Mart gains us critical items for Amelia, such as a car seat. Road trips rule when driving 360 miles across Alaska. I have not been to Fairbanks. On our way out of town, we stop to gas up.

Cindy glances at the headlines of the daily paper: Fairbanks Fires. Evacuations. "Kat, have you seen this?"

I shake my head and grasp the paper to read the details of what is going on. "It can't be that bad," I say, determined and stubborn. "We have to check it out."

The first 200 miles up to Fairbanks are gorgeous. It is likely the last 150 miles are the same, but visibility is below a quarter mile from thick smoke.

"Maybe we should have waited a couple days," Cindy says.

Classes start in a couple of days, and we have a lot to do to get ready.

"Life waits for no one. It'll be better in Fairbanks," I say.

I should know by now that ignorant optimism isn't always the best planning strategy. In Alaska that year, 4.7 million acres of forest burn—the third-worst fire year in the state's history. The EPA issues a hazardous air quality warning for five days, cautioning people to avoid outdoor exertion and keep kids inside. Welcome to Fairbanks.

We first live in campus housing, which has the convenience of running water. That, combined with automatic electric heat, feels way too upscale for me. As Cindy predicted, I move us into a series of cabins that have woodstoves and either no running water or water pumped in by truck to an underground storage tank. But all of them still have the luxury of electricity, quite the novelty after the hard-won, intermittent power available at camp.

▸CYCLES OF GRIEF

FAIRBANKS, ALASKA | 2004–2007

Between grief and nothing I will take grief.

—WILLIAM FAULKNER

The first years after Dave's death I survive, stuck in denial, numbness, avoidance, and shame. My grieving process borders on bipolar. I have weeks of intense productivity at school and work followed by weeks of remorse, unforgiving depression, and isolation. Shame holds my soul prisoner. Flashbacks of Madi's death recur at regular intervals and with increased intensity during the months of her birth and death.

I stay true to a path leading to a meaningful life with Amelia. I strive every day to rise above the shadow of mourning to parent with happy devotion. The life sparkling in her eyes pulls me away from despair and into the present moment. She makes it easy to build a future and generate new memories. Amelia's well-being takes priority. Her spunky and creative personality grows by the day, and I know how fortunate I am to have such a perfect young girl to call my daughter.

Lacking a heartfelt dream to work towards, I focus on achieving practical milestones. My degree is a means to an end and a way to put one foot in front of the other. I get my Emergency Medical Technician I, II, and III certifications to arm myself with knowledge for the next time disaster strikes. I work toward my bachelor's degree. I create an interdisciplinary degree program in renewable energy engineering that combines computational physics and electrical and mechanical engineering with renewable energy modeling. I overachieve to compensate for my perceived failures.

I date random men and leave a trail of relationship chaos as my heart can never commit. Well-meaning men want to love and help Amelia and me. I try to go along with it, hoping my heart will come back to life, but then it shuts down, leaving them feeling used. I even get engaged to a wonderful, patient man who loves and accepts Amelia. He proposes on a hunting trip in the Brooks Range. Talk about a dream come true. But I destroy that relationship too, feeling I don't deserve a new dream yet.

One old dream I can pursue is being a pilot. This dream began when reading *Arctic Daughter* at age ten, but I set it aside because Dave didn't trust small, single-engine airplanes. In Kotzebue, flying will allow me to peruse river bluffs and spot mammoth ivory from above. Now it was time to pursue my license. I go home to stay with Mom in Minneapolis and work on it during a two-month stay.

My first time soloing is in a Cessna 172 in the Anoka County Airport in Minneapolis in 2007. I have the required sixteen hours of flight time, and the goal is for me to take a forty-minute solo flight. Ten minutes away from the airport, I hear a loud bang and feel rattling in the engine. Not being versed in airplane mechanics, I come close to peeing my pants. I turn the plane around, hoping I can make it back to the airport. Knowing I lack sufficient skill, I don't want to attempt an emergency landing on my first solo flight. I execute the practiced diligence in safe piloting by planning out emergency procedures and landings. I land back at the Anoka Airport. The flight school mechanics find a cracked piston. The next day I am back in the air, flying above the clouds practicing slow flight maneuvers. Rip that Band-Aid off.

It only requires forty hours of flight time to get your license, and that's what I do. I absorb the material, and the written exams are easy for me. With minimal actual flight time, the practical exam is stressful, but I perform the required flight maneuvers on the first try and get my license.

A float rating requires a ten-hour flying-time endorsement by a certified float-rating instructor. In Fairbanks, I get my float rating, which qualifies me to take off and land in water. This is my favorite type of flying. I practice touch-and-goes at a seaplane base in Fairbanks with Amelia seat-belted in the back. We can take the airplane up and find anywhere to land. There are lakes everywhere of sufficient length for landing and taking off. I love learning how to read the waves and know what the wind is doing based on how the water looks from high above.

Eager to surround myself with aviation, I work as a ramp agent at an airline called Warbelow's that serves Interior Alaska villages. I load and unload airplanes. I want to fly as a commercial pilot. Being around airplanes and learning about the business is important. I am promoted to the dispatch office and work as a Part 135 dispatcher. I attend a six-week program in Galena, Alaska, to become a Part 121 dispatcher, which enables me to dispatch for large airlines such as Alaska Airlines.

While in Galena, I meet Captain Bill and his wife, Sue, who take Amelia and me under their wings. Bill lands me a job at Frontier Airlines. We all become close friends for many years.

After working as a dispatcher, I see how difficult it is for the pilots. They have no regular schedules. When they are grounded because of weather, they don't get paid. There are long layovers they have no control over. It is plain that this is not a solution for me with a young child.

Cassie comes up to Fairbanks to stay with Amelia and me for the summer. Cassie is still in high school and having this solo time with her is a gift. She learns how to drive in our bright-yellow jeep with a stick shift. We take the top off, put Amelia in a car seat in the back, and drive through the backroads of Gold Stream Valley. Amelia urges Cassie to drive through the mud puddles as fast as she can. Cassie and Amelia hang out while I work and attend classes. Amelia is lucky to have such phenomenal aunties.

I float from one achievement to the next. Occasionally I break out of my self-diagnosed bipolar grief cycle, move toward acceptance, and make a new plan for life. I search for meaning in what happened. Still, the ups and downs around key anniversaries continue to destroy anything positive in our lives. It is difficult to gift yourself with the time to grieve, but at some point, I will have to. I don't let go of the shared dream Dave and I built, but I need to redefine a few of its elements.

▸HOME AGAIN

KOBUK LAKE, ALASKA | 2008

The clearest way into the Universe
is through a forest wilderness.

—JOHN MUIR

Landing back in Kotzebue, a sudden feeling of excitement rushes through me. My body knows I am closing in on home. On the flight over, I can see the expansive north shore of Kobuk Lake, and if I squint hard enough, I can almost make out our cabin. Amelia, now four-years-old, has her own airplane seat. Never being one to sleep on airplanes, she is wide awake and ready to get off the plane.

It will be a busy and difficult day. Things never come easy in keeping equipment running above the Arctic Circle. The boat is going back in the water for the first time this year. I last parked our old Dodge truck a half mile from the airport. Rather than wait at the airport to visit with old friends, Amelia and I walk to get the truck started. I cross my fingers, hoping the engine turns over. Nothing. I take out the jumper cables from behind the seat and open the hood. After a couple of minutes, Dickie Moto pulls over. He says hi to Amelia, who remembers him. Together, we get the truck started, and I go back to the airport to get our six totes of supplies for the month ahead.

The next chore is to get the boat in the water. This easy task is challenging with Amelia. It is a gorgeous mid-July day. The sun is high in a clear blue sky, and it will remain light out around the clock for a couple more weeks. A few preventative chores can keep the outboard running longer. I change the spark plugs and the oil on the lower unit while the boat is out of the water. Amelia helps by distributing tools around the ground and making mud pies. With summer comes mosquitoes, and I douse us good with as much deet as I can find. My parenting can come into question later, when she isn't being threatened with endless swollen, itchy welts.

I sit Amelia in the truck as I back our boat into the protected lagoon behind Kotzebue. Telling Amelia to sit down in the truck seat, I run out back to jump onto the boat. In my mind, many things happen to Amelia while I am stuck on the boat parking it: Amelia falls off the seat and hits her head. Amelia puts something in her mouth and chokes. Amelia somehow turns the truck on and puts it in neutral; it rolls into the water, and she drowns. I stop. My plan will not cut it.

I get back into the truck to give her a great big hug and reevaluate. "Amelia, how would you like to go for a short boat ride?"

How are we going to do this? I already have my hip boots on, but the water is too deep to walk out and put her into the boat. If I had my chest waders from camp, I could make that work. I sit in the truck for about twenty minutes, thinking through my options, when along comes Uncle Lee McClain. Uncle Lee is a local bone hunter, ivory carver, knife maker, and gunsmith who loves to spend his summers in his inflatable raft scouring the beaches for mammoth teeth and other items of interest. He is Alaskan to the core. While not a blood relation, Amelia has her Uncle Lee wrapped around her little finger, and the two of them are like peas in a pod. Lee already has plans to teach Amelia to shoot and has her first .22 ready.

"Need help?" Lee says.

Grateful nearly to tears, I run over and give him a big hug of hello. "I'd love some!" I say.

He jumps into the truck with Amelia next to him. "Get on in that boat," he calls out.

I climb on the back of the truck to jump over onto the bow. The high stern of the Olympic always makes getting on and off a gymnastic feat. I walk with care on the small ledge of the boat cabin before jumping into the back of the boat. Lee and I have put enough boats in the water to know this routine well and don't have to communicate. I unlock the outboard and lower it into the water, prime the pump on the fuel hose, choke it, cross my fingers, and turn the key. Success at last. We let it warm up for a few minutes, making sure it is operating as it should. Lee gives me a thumbs up, I nod, and he backs up a few more feet. The boat comes off the trailer, gliding backward into the deeper water of the lagoon. The calm day has blessed us with flat water. Knowing Amelia is in good company, I take the boat out in a wide circle, listening for any potential problems. I would rather find them now than with Amelia twenty miles out of town. Satisfied, I circle back to the lagoon and throw out the rear anchor. I pull in sideways to the beach and put the front anchor down on shore. I need the rear of the boat to be close to the beach, so I can pump in gas from the drum in the back of our Dodge. I jump out of the boat and run up to Amelia, who jumps up hoping to get into the boat.

"Hey, Amelia Bedelia, ready to go on a boat ride?"

Amelia jumps up and down in response.

"You gonna be okay out there?" There is a lot more to Lee's question than one would think. He was close to Dave and knows how hard it will be to go home to an empty house.

"Thanks. We'll make it work. It's great to be home."

He raises his eyebrows. Without my dad here, Lee steps into that role "I know when you're lying," he says. "The color of your eyes change depending on if you are happy or sad. Right now, they sure aren't happy eyes."

"Seriously," I continue. "We need to face things. Amelia and I will take our time. If I need anything, I will call."

Shaking his head he lifts in shoulders in surrender.

"Thank you so much for your help," I say.

"No sweat," he says, giving Amelia a kiss on the cheek before hopping back in his own truck to leave.

"Well, Amelia, time to go?" I ask.

Amelia nods her head in excitement.

She plays on the beach picking up rocks as I put our six totes into the boat and pump gas. I load into the boat twenty gallons of gas in jerry jugs for the four-wheeler and generator, a twenty-pound propane tank for our oven, and a heavy thirty-gallon water container. Amelia and I run to the grocery store for a few supplies, like sandwich material and juice for the boat ride home. I also grab perishables I didn't pack in Fairbanks, including cheese, milk, eggs, and butter. Oh yeah, and bug spray. Getting to the cash register, it rings up at $105.20.

"What?" I ask.

My job as a ramp agent at Warbelow's Air Service pays fourteen dollars an hour. That bit of food is equivalent to an eight-hour workday. Ouch! I forgot how expensive things are in Kotzebue.

I place Amelia in her boat seat, jump out to grab the front anchor and push the rear end of the boat out, then jump back in to start the outboard to let it warm up again. I run to the back of the boat and pull up on the rear anchor, taking us out to the deeper water. I can now put the lower unit deeper in the water as I angle us toward the bridge that marks the way out of the lagoon and into Kobuk Lake.

Easing forward on the throttle, Amelia and I both yell "Wahoo!" as the boat picks up speed and gets up "on step," where it glides with the least amount of drag across the water surface.

With a loaded boat, our definition of speed is likely not that fast, but it feels like we are flying a million miles an hour as the adrenaline pours into us both. We are back in our boat, together, and heading toward our home, the place we love more than any other. I don't allow myself to feel sadness that those we love most in the world are no longer there waiting to greet us, that only their crosses are.

"Wahoo!" I yell out again, smiling big at Amelia.

"Scooby-dooby-doo!" she replies with equal enthusiasm—an enthusiasm that will chase away any ghosts.

There isn't room for death and life in this boat. I have to choose one, and it isn't any contest (see fig. 39).

►ACHIEVE

FAIRBANKS, ALASKA | 2008

We do not write in order to be understood;
we write in order to understand.

—C. DAY-LEWIS

"Katherine Keith!" The dean of the University of Alaska Fairbanks calls out my name.

My hands clench in nervous anticipation under the folds of my black robe. I keep my head down to ensure my feet go one step in front of the other. The square graduation cap hides my teary eyes from onlookers.

"Recipient of the 2008 Gray S. Tilly Memorial Award and one of eighty nationwide recipients of the Morris K. Udall Foundation Scholarship," he continues.

We did it. Today, I graduate college. My mom flew up from Minnesota to be here.

The dean continues, "Katherine and her husband built a home and started a family while living a subsistence lifestyle. The deaths of her husband and eldest child turned her life in a different direction. Keith saw global events risking the ecosystem around her, and she wanted to make a difference. She is graduating with an interdisciplinary degree in renewable energy engineering and a minor in computational physics. She plans to pursue a graduate degree in power system engineering and use her education to help create sustainable communities and resolve energy challenges."

I square up my shoulders, hold my head up high, and look straight toward the podium and my diploma. My stride, no longer hesitant, lengthens. I bounce up the stairs to shake the hand of the dean. Raw joy courses through me. Amelia, five-years-old, isn't likely to remember this moment. More than any other, walking down this aisle is my biggest achievement. I do this for her. She needs a mom to be proud of and to know that she can do anything she sets her mind to. I bite my lip so as not to cry. Resolve courses through me—the same grit that sustained me every day since I started classes, or rather, every day of my life. Amelia will have a life she can build on and do anything she puts her heart into. Nothing will hold her back. My single-minded determination on this matter has only escalated through the years.

Life took away a lot from us. To fight back, I take it back and give it all to her. That is my purpose now. Damn fate. Amelia will live to the fullest. The choices, love, options, trials, and tribulations—hers for the dreaming, reaching, and even falling. (Less falling preferred.) When she falls, it should be epic. Good falls, worth telling about, always are. She will have me to show her how to stand up again, dream again, and live again. It doesn't matter where we have been, only that Amelia and I have a future to embark on together.

►RESILIENCE

PALMER, ALASKA | 2008

---

*When you want something, all the universe
conspires in helping you to achieve it.*

—PAULO COELHO

After graduation, my career takes off in a positive direction. Energy engineering work keeps me busy and, through different jobs and ventures, I work on multiple projects all across the state. Grief still follows me home like a lost and hungry puppy. How long does it take to get over loss? Haven't I resolved this yet? Time to get more proactive about it. I have the attitude to get over it but haven't done the work. I need to transform grief. Inspiration is easy, but follow-through is a bitch of an uphill climb.

Endurance racing becomes a tool for recovery and helps me to establish healthy goals. Training allows me to say yes to life's positive opportunities. I can get up and run, bike, or swim and am one step closer to being in charge of life.

Physical challenges reconnect me to my body. I can feel my body instead of remaining mired in the numb hollowness I accept as normal. The exertion that racing demands makes me put one foot in front of the other. I am no longer a passive bystander in my life but an active and driven athlete. The distinction wakes me up and reminds me who I am—I am more than my grief, more than my loss, more than my shame. I race as I do with most things in life: at full speed. I complete my first sprint-distance triathlon in 2008.

As I cross the finish line, I am sold on what a triathlon can do for a healing journey. It fills me with hope again. I next do an Olympic-distance triathlon, then a half-Ironman, until I find my home in the full-distance Ironman.

An assistant professor position with the University of Alaska, running their Renewable Energy Certificate program, brings me to Palmer, Alaska, a small town just outside Anchorage, with a view of the Chugach Mountains. Cindy decides to move back up to Alaska to join us in Palmer. I dream again. Dreaming of new adventures, dog mushing, mountain climbing, camp, and the unexplored wilderness I can now share with Amelia.

I train for my first full Ironman event, the Silverman in Henderson, Nevada, held on the six-year anniversary of Dave's death. I sign up for the race with the clear intention of turning away from being a victim of circumstance and toward seizing control over what I want to do with my future.

Training for this race is a way for me to process my grief. The two years of intense physical training leading up to the Silverman support a lot of emotional healing. Past finishers report the event to be brutal, with severe hills and intense heat that includes a 2.4-mile swim, a 112-mile bike ride, and a 26.2-mile run.

It is difficult to train for an Ironman as a single parent. I spend five hours a day on the stationary bike inside the house watching movies with Amelia and take long runs on a treadmill close by her so we can talk. Most mornings I wake up early to keep my training from interfering with family life. Every Ironman athlete knows that separating our training regime from daily life and family is impossible. Ironman training requires tremendous sacrifice of families. It influences life year-round, dictating everything—what you eat, what you do for fun, what you want to talk about, and what you want to wear. Even days when you're not training are active rest days where you focus on recovery. We like to talk about heart rates, nutrition, the latest gear, and our training plan for the week. Our poor families.

Ironman training regimens consume an average of thirty hours each week. On top of which is food preparation, traveling to train, and other organizational activities. I begin with books that talk about training routines, and I sketch out my training plans. I make a lot of mistakes. My regular program includes running four days a week, biking four days a week, swimming three days a week, and one strength session.

The uninterrupted time, lost in thought, is voluntary for me. I distract myself through audiobooks and podcasts if I don't want to be in my head. But I enjoy my company enough that the meditational space endurance activities provide gives me a lot of balance to check in on my inner world.

Traveling to the Silverman racecourse includes a bizarre juxtaposition flying into Las Vegas from Alaska, then traveling to the scenic Lake Mead National Recreational Area. The swim begins at Boulder Beach and the warm water is crystal clear. I manage the swim without inhaling gallons of water and arrive at T1, the first transition area, in good spirits.

The bike section is notorious for its hills, but I have been training for this. Still, I am unprepared for the 8,500 feet of total elevation gain. The course follows along the west and north shores of Lake Mead before heading back into Henderson. On the bike, I am so nauseous from heat and exertion that I can't eat my race-day nutrition, leaving me weak. Nothing is flat. All I can focus on is getting to the next aid station where I can pour water over my head, hoping to cool down. There is no shade out on this high desert, and the temperatures are rising close to ninety degrees Fahrenheit. I cry in frustration over my discomfort and my inability to thrive. The tears transition to those of anger, shame, and grief over having my loved ones ripped away from me so soon. Suffering is universal; what differs is the trigger. I take the anger and pour it into my legs, driving away my soul's pain with every climb.

By the time I reach the bike transition area, T2, my body spasms in pain. My neck aches from the bike handlebars, welts on my neck are raw from my wetsuit and sunburn, and sand makes it into my bike shoes, creating blisters on my feet. My quads and hamstrings are jelly. It is time to put on my sneakers to start a 26.2-mile run. I fall off the bike, and I can't walk.

The crowd cheers me on, shouting out encouragement. "You can do this! You got this! Keep it up! You're my hero!"

Meanwhile, I waddle like an elderly Donald Duck. But the words penetrate through the pain in both my body and my soul. I absorb the crowd's support, and it fuels my legs to take one foot and put it in front of the other—one baby-step at a time, like the previous six years.

This crawling, hesitant pace isn't enough for me anymore—not for this race, not for my life. Instead, I want to live. Putting one foot in front of the other isn't enough. I want to fly. I run. It does not look like flying—still more like a Donald Duck shuffle—but inside I soar free. I leave behind my broken heart and replace it with the encouraging words of random strangers.

Mile after mile I recall, for the first time ever, happy memories of Dave and Madi—times when we were all together, and times when Amelia, Dave, Alan, and I were out in the boat, exploring the world with nothing but time and each other. These memories replace the tragedy. The running gives me the resilience to feel the joy of these memories rather than the pain of their absence.

A couple of miles from the finish, I run by a little girl who shouts out, "You are an Ironwoman!"

Her words persist through my physical discomfort.

As I cross the finish line, the announcers say, "Katherine, you are an *Ironman!*"

My body may be battered, but I am still flying.

There was no turning back, and I commit to race one Ironman per year to help me keep that focus and keep me saying "Yes!" I choose every day to live to the fullest. Resilience is power, is freedom (see fig. 40).

▸BUDDHA AND THE SKY

KOTZEBUE, ALASKA | 2012

Nowhere else in nature—not in the comings and goings of the birds, the blossoming of trees, nor the arrival of the rains—do we find a more reliable environmental reality in which to frame the drama of life than the celestial backdrop.

—ANTHONY AVENI,
SKYWATCHERS OF ANCIENT MEXICO

I enjoy visiting Kotzebue during long stays out at camp and am eager to move back home. I have barriers to moving—practical ones as well as psychological ones. Kotzebue has taken a lot from me, although it has given back. Part of me doesn't want Amelia back there, exposed to the risks of life above the Arctic Circle. Overall, I fear the ultimate cost of reinvesting in a life there.

Despite my reticence, Kotzebue was, and is, my home. I've been working as an energy engineer for a design firm, WHPacific, and the company has me establish a local office in Kotzebue. Amelia is in third grade when we move back to Kotzebue in March 2012. Cindy comes up to to work for a while.

In Kotzebue, there is no swimming pool for Ironman training, only one road to run, and no roads to ride a triathlon bike on. My training will be all indoors. On weekends, Cindy, Amelia, and I cruise out to camp whenever weather permits.

I want to dream again. Time to change, even if it seems like a step forward over a cliff when I know I can't fly. Restless, I walk down the beach and gaze at the moon. The universe reveals a lesson. The moon has a beautiful rainbow halo, adding a touch of intrigue and harmony to the black beyond. Clouds blanket the sky, and my heart falls at the lack of stars. Within the hour, cloud cover shifts to the west, revealing the moon while dissipating the rainbow halo. The stunning halo needs cloud cover to contrast its loveliness.

I want my heart, body, and spirit to be whole—to be free from suffering, as I once hoped for out in the dog yard of the Itens. I want to come full circle to be a bodhisattva. How can I ever help anybody else if I am lost? I have earmarked many Thich Nhat Hanh books. The breathing meditations he offers give hope that the worst mental cancer can improve through simple and dedicated practice. "Breathing in, I smile. Breathing out, I release. Breathing in, dwelling in the present moment. Breathing out, it is a wonderful moment." Yes, Thich Nhat Hanh, thanks to you, it is a wonderful moment.

I look to a night sky full of magic. The moon, above the horizon, circles twenty-four hours a day. The clear night sky brings alive the mysteries of the stars. Our ancient ancestors looked to the stars for their source of truth. I see truth in stars in the present moment. Judgment of right or wrong doesn't exist when you bare your soul in total vulnerability to look, full of wonder, up at the stars. I find refuge in the night sky. Wake up heart!

The celestial spheres intrigued eons of civilizations with their mystery, beauty, and power. Shamans, chiefs, and kings leveraged their connection to the sky above us to rise over their circumstances, raise the stature of their people, and connect to the afterlife. My fascination with the ancient sky reaches back twenty years. As a child sitting at the campfire with my dad toasting marshmallows, we would look up to talk about the constellations. The lights we see and the skies we watch create a window to the gods. The stage that the sky sets, with its many layers, weaves a story so complex yet so simple we humans can't help but be in utter awe. From Mesoamerica, to the Forbidden City of Beijing, to ancient Egypt, to the Celts of Ireland, the ancient peoples all knew a common supernatural truth. We are not islands unto ourselves. We are part of a greater mystery called life. That our strand in the web of life is but one part of a beautiful whole. The light I shine is one among a tapestry of stars. The stars own my adoration and respect.

The mystery of the stars weaves a tapestry with the simple rules of Buddhism. Together they form a strong cord, which I consider my lifeline. I have been that archeologist who lifts a potsherd out of soil where it lay hidden for centuries. What is the story behind that potsherd? How old is it? Where does it originate from? Who made it? How did they create it? What were they thinking? Who did they worship when their lives were dark as night with no hope? Did they follow rules similar to that of a Buddhist? Did they look up and ask the moon to help guide them? I can hold that potsherd and lose myself for hours in the imaginative pathways of my mind.

The rules of cosmic order sync with the Eightfold Path, the Four Noble Truths, and the Six Perfections. If I follow the laws of nature, follow the cosmic order of things, I shall be back on the path of the bodhisattva. If my actions are in alignment with nature, how can I go astray? Maybe I am oversimplifying things.

There is a cosmic order to things. Dr. E. C. Krupp, author of *Echoes of the Ancient Skies*, states that, "What we see in the lights overhead is the itinerary of cosmic order. Because it governs everything, it is reflected in the entire world. It is the core of our consciousness. It defines what is sacred and makes the sky the domain of gods."

May the inner stillness and serenity found among the stars grow within your soul. I fall asleep, wake up to a new day, and begin again. Rinse. Repeat.

▸SHAMAN

KOTZEBUE, ALASKA | 2015

The snow goose need not bathe to make itself white.
Neither need you do anything but be yourself.

—LAO TZU

After the close call with Loki and scratching in the 2015 Iditarod, I have deep soul-searching to do. It has been ten years since I lost Dave and Madi; twenty since the fateful sun dance and remembrance of abuse. I have moved on with building a new dream for myself and my family. How does their loss still cripple me? I need to face it more head on. Time to declare war on mourning. I have tried therapy, Ironman races, dog races—all methods to let go of the toxic buildup. Still it bubbles up in my weakest moments. Being bitter about life's randomness, I turned my back on spiritual practices. Perhaps now is the time to return.

What way is the right way? The Eightfold Path, the Ten Commandments, or do I make my own path? My diverse spiritual wanderings have led me from one end of the spectrum to the other. I alone am responsible for my spiritual growth and destiny. I can be a victim or an advocate for my life and the lives of those I love. Not a hard decision to make.

Since I was a child, shamanic traditions have long called out as a path of evidence-based inquiry into the spiritual foundations of our present lives and the lives of our ancestors. Shamanism is not a religion or faith, but a knowing. Without a mechanism for proper training, I explored Celtic shamanism as a teenager then later pursued understanding of Native American practices with tribes in New Mexico and Arizona. While none of these cultural practices seemed to be a good fit, it formed the basis of my spiritual practice. In searching for meaning, I traveled all over the United States finding the wild and free in our great country. I took myself to remote locations, hungry for something. After losing Dave and Madi, my spiritual search went on the back burner while I struggled with grief in a more mundane way.

Research indicates that shamans are wounded healers, or they may inherit the healing gift from their shaman ancestors. Tibetan shamans are hereditary but skip a generation. The Inuit of Greenland get left on the ice for days with no clothes or food to see if they survive. Sometimes dreams call to shamans who follow their dream through initiatory practices. Some places let you pay a master shaman to provide initiation experiences to see what happens.

There is a loss of knowledge worldwide. Elders are not available to youth as they once were. In generations past, the Inuit elders in Hudson Bay knew people who had starved because they couldn't find caribou. The shamans would use divination to find answers to such pragmatic questions. They would take a caribou shoulder blade and read it, like a map, to determine location of game. I don't plan on reading the shoulder blades of dead animals, but there is something in the method that has lasted thousands of years and spanned the globe.

Shamans in northwest Alaska have historically created both real benefit and real harm. Not all shamans want to help others. Sorcerers of the past longed for power, cursed their neighbors, and warred with nearby villages. When missionaries came in the mid-1900s, indigenous practices such as drumming and dancing were considered devil worship and banned. They took away all drums—the heartbeat of a culture, stolen in a decade.

Core Shamanism, founded by the late Michael Harner, brings together universal, near universal, and common practices making it well-suited to contemporary practitioners.

Practicing the path of a shaman, I listen to the beat of the drum traveling around non-ordinary reality, questing to find answers to this puzzling life. With every initiation, deep revelations pour forth. Carlos Castaneda was onto something. Profound awareness enters my being. The traumas embedded in my soul release their grip. I forgive others and forgive myself. The core of my being understands that enlightenment is no longer my goal. This life is not about helping me for my benefit. It is about easing the pain and suffering of others. The shamanic path has the same endgame as a bodhisattva, where enlightenment is a mere side effect. I do not want to use any mind-altering substances. I want the authentic experience—hard-earned through training.

Core shamanism methods use only a drum or rattle to induce theta brain waves (four to seven beats per second), the most effective for altering consciousness. The theta ranges cause the brain waves to entrain and to fall in sync with the beat of the drum. Shamans need to develop the discipline to have one foot in each reality and be in either when needed.

I find an inner knowing about life and our purpose here. A shaman treats everything with great respect, sees and knows with the heart, and makes the impossible possible. I won't allow myself to be inauthentic again. I will be true, damn the consequences.

▸YUKON QUEST

WHITEHORSE, CANADA | 2017

The vast and empty swath of land comprising Alaska's Interior and Canada's Yukon Territory is reserved for the rugged and the romantic, the bold, the independent and the centered self, not the self-centered. It is the land of dreamers and of rich traditions. This is a place the intrepid choose in winter. They do not fear temperatures dropping to -50 Fahrenheit. For the strong minded the Far North's extremes offer an affirmation that they are alive. For the weak-minded, it is the wrong place to be.

—LEW FREEDMAN, *YUKON QUEST*

The 2017 Yukon Quest race begins in Whitehorse, Yukon. This race trail runs one thousand miles across northern Alaska and the Yukon Territory. Most mushers consider it the toughest sled dog race in the world. Compared to the Iditarod, the Yukon Quest has many more summits to climb, half the checkpoints, and far colder temperatures. The motto of the Quest is, Survive First, Race Second.

My preparation began ten years ago in Fairbanks, when I first heard of its existence while working at Chena Hot Springs on geothermal energy projects. The Yukon Quest trail passes right alongside the property at Chena, so the race brings a sense of wonder of what unexplored mysteries lie beyond the boundaries of what is already a remote location. Chena Hot Springs is the end of the road for cars. A paved road extends sixty miles from Fairbanks and dead-ends at the hot springs. For mushers, that is where it all begins. That is all my wanderlust needs to take root, although I had no long-distance racing experience, or any real mushing experience, at that point.

Looking out over the hills, I dream about the Far North wilderness mushers venture into. I want to experience that for myself. The history of the trail is fascinating. It follows old gold-mining and mail-delivery routes opened in the late 1800s by miners, trappers, and mail carriers. In 1984 they ran the first Quest. Its purpose was "to offer an experience that reflects the spirit and perseverance of the pioneers who discovered themselves in their wild search for adventure, glory, and wealth in the Frozen North" and "to recognize and promote the spirit that compels one to live in the Great North Land, an international spirit that knows no governmental boundaries, and to bring public attention to the historic role of the Arctic Trail in the development of the North Country, and the people and animals that strove to meet its challenge."

The Yukon Quest is infamous for extreme cold and desolate landscapes with endless days of solitude. There are four notorious summits: King Solomon's Dome, American, Eagle, and Rosebud. The Yukon River has mazes of broken-up jumble ice that lasts for miles. One stretch of trail from Pelly Crossing checkpoint to Dawson is two hundred miles long. The enthusiasm for the trail does nothing to reduce my outright fear in the months leading up to the race. I have nightmares of the race, and the preparations for it haunt my waking and sleeping hours.

In *Yukon Quest: The History of the World's Toughest Sled Dog Race*, Lew Freedman writes, "There will come a time and a place along the trail when the body is weakening, the cold is penetrating to the bones, visibility is non-existent because of blowing snow, when the dogs and musher would prefer to lie down in the night. At such a time, the musher must reach down to find out if he has the right stuff." This is the source of my massive feeling of unease. I stared down my demons on thousands of miles of lonely trail leading up to this point, and think I have what it takes.

Writer John Schandelmeier said, "The Quest trail demands the highest caliber of skill and readiness from mushers and their teams. Many who start don't make it to the finish."

I know what I am getting into. Perfect. I am hungry for that connection found when driving yourself to the edge of what most people consider sane. Or maybe I am overconfident.

Four weeks before the Iditarod, the Yukon Quest runs from Whitehorse to Fairbanks, alternating direction every year. This means that the dogs and I will run in two different thousand-mile dogsled races with little more than a two-week break between. I have the company of Nina Schwinghammer and her mechanically inclined fiancé, Alan Spangler. They are working as handlers to support the race by driving a truck two thousand miles to pick up any dropped dogs and clean up the straw and leftover food after we leave the checkpoints.

I have a great team of dogs snuggling in their straw-filled boxes in a sixteen-foot toy hauler. My main leaders are Blondie, Joy, Katherine, and Giant. All four of them have significant racing experience. Joy is the only one who has completed multiple thousand-mile races with me. The team includes four brothers: Flash, Shadow, Stark, and Loki who came back strong from the 2015 Iditarod. To fill out the twelve-dog team, I also have Neo, the oldest gal on the team at six years old.

It is amazing that no matter how prepared you are going into race week, there are always last-minute details that somehow create a disproportionate amount of stress. If left behind, little things like extra AA batteries, zip ties for the sled banners, or toenail clippers for the dogs can create massive problems. Using checklists is a great "type A" way to eliminate most disasters. But there is always something that ends up making me cry out, "My race is ruined!"

Race day is here. I wake up and fill my coffee and hot water thermoses. Nina, Alan, and I look for the entrance to the musher parking and get settled in. Three hours until lift off, I put on my parka. It is about ten below and I don't want to get cold before heading out. I zip up my beloved $800 can't-live-without Arc'teryx jacket, when—*snap!*—the zipper breaks. I am in disbelief. I have to leave in three hours and have a useless parka I can't zip, and now I will freeze in the frigid Far North of the Quest.

"My race is ruined!" I yell while crying.

I always seem to cry at race start lines. I have to go ten days without talking to Amelia. I get torn up knowing how nervous and scared she will be. She won't be able to hear my voice. I cry in the back of the trailer, hoping no one comes in and sees me. I'm panicking over this zipper and Amelia and crying. Great. This is where having resilient friends, family, and handlers around you can make or break your race experience.

"How about I go over to the local ski shop and get a replacement," Alan says.

In my mind, I determine there is no way they will have the exact one. It won't suffice, and even if it does, it will cost $1,000. I have no choice. The biggest rule of thumb for Arctic travel is that you *always* test your gear. I am heading out for ten days with my main piece of clothing untested. Having no available car, Alan physically runs to the store one mile away and begins the shopping process. They don't have the same style or anything close to it. Arc'teryx designed a new layer system for improved flexibility, and I have no clue as to its effectiveness. I know what works for me. Pretty much just Arc'teryx Gore-Tex outer layers, wool inner layers, and Arc'teryx synthetic down. Although the zipper failed me, I trust it keep me dry and warm. Alan runs the mile back to the dog truck so I can try on what he found. They don't fit.

We are now at T-minus-2 hours, and you guessed it: "My race is ruined!" I cry on the phone to Mom. I prefer to be alone in the prerace hours. I know and accept that I am irrational and work to minimize the fallout on poor innocent bystanders. Nina and Alan are unfortunate, being stuck with me.

Alan runs back, another mile, to shop around for new sizes and styles. He returns with another option, and it fits! The new gear is lighter, warmer, and more comfortable. Despite costing loads, the new gear might save my race. Mushers need a lot of coat pockets. We stuff everything we don't want to lose or that can't freeze into them. It is easy to get lazy and want to keep your survival gear in a bag on the sled, but if you fall off of it during the race at forty degrees below zero, that could pose a problem. I fill my pockets with lighters, two 5-Hour Energy shots, a pocketknife, a GPS, hand warmers, backup contact lenses, eye drops, a headlamp, a headlamp battery, etc.

T-minus-1.5 hours. The next hurdle is to put on new plastic—my biggest racing obstacle. No matter what I do, putting on new sled-runner plastic always results in crisis. You want to wait until race morning so the plastic doesn't get damaged in the trailer before the start. This time, the company who sells the runners neglected to drill holes into the hard plastic. We can't secure them to the nine-foot sled runners.

"My race is ruined!" I cry out again.

At that moment, Tyrell Seavey comes up to say hi. A racer himself, Tyrell is the brother of Dallas Seavey, four-time Iditarod champion, and no a stranger to race-start issues. To make me feel better, he tells me of a time when Dallas ran the Denali Doubles sled dog race.

"My brother drives up from his home in Wasilla, has his dogs harnessed and sled out. About one hour before race start, he realizes he forgot one important piece of gear: his gang line. Most people give up at that point. Not Dallas. Dallas nonchalantly puts a gang line together with a rope he finds in the back of the truck. Despite having young dogs, known for chewing, he takes off on time. Plus, Dallas wins the race. His cool temperament proved to be an asset."

I take the hint: breathe, and work to stay calm. Tyrell and Alan take over working on the sled plastic by finding a drill and bit from somewhere. We go through all the plastic and find that none of it has holes. This means that they also screwed up all the plastic in my drop bags along the trail. I have to drill out whatever plastic I can find in the trailer and carry it with me as I won't be able to do so on the trail.

T-minus-1 hour. I pack the sled. Nina and I harness the dogs. It's time to put booties on each of their paws. I have on all my gear and load my pockets with critical items. People want to laugh, talk, and share in the excitement of the trail ahead. I sneak away into the front of the truck to call Amelia to say goodbye because it is time to hand my phone over to Nina—the Yukon Quest board does not allow two-way communication devices on the trail. Amelia is worried, but she doesn't let me hear it in her voice. She is used to the routine from the Iditarod, but the unfamiliarity of the Yukon Quest trail creates uncertainty.

We are now at the starting line. I have Blondie and Joy in lead to get us to the first checkpoint, Braeburn, which is one hundred miles away. I relax, knowing I can't do any more to be ready. My race is not ruined.

A thousand miles of brand-new trail stretches out ahead of me, taking me to places I have only read and dreamed about. The dogs are frenzied with excitement, jerking on the line trying to pull the sled loose, wagging their tails, and barking. It is thrilling and contagious. They know we are ready to go.

The timekeeper says, "Go!"

I pull the hooks, volunteers let go of my sled, and we fly down the trail. I leave Whitehorse behind with a sigh of relief and a sense of excitement, knowing that an uncharted territory lies in store for the dogs and me.

Fifteen miles into the race, on the way to Braeburn, is the first trail crux. There is open water on the Takhini River, so the trail needs to go overland on a new trail. We pass through trees and prepare to drop onto the river in the next few miles. Soon I hear dog teams stopped ahead of me. The wooded trail is too narrow to attempt passing. The dogs are riled up, barking, and jerking. Needing to see what the problem is, I find a small tree to wrap my hook around and walk up to talk to the musher in front of me while keeping an eye on my team. Together we figure out what is going on.

The trail ahead zigzags with four extreme 90-degree turns within twenty feet of each other. The last of these is a left turn with a sheer three-hundred-foot drop-off to the right. To make matters interesting, this left-corner turn also has trees. Right now, a sled is stuck to one of them, and the musher is working to free it, with all dogs jerking, while trying to not fall over the edge.

The priority for mushers is the safety of their own dog team, but we always assist others in crisis situations, and this is one of those times. With help, the first team breaks loose and careens down the extreme downhill trail. Sebastian, a rookie Quest musher, is next, but his team is overexcited. As he pulls his hook to get under way, his sled wraps on a tree that tips it. He frees the sled, tips it on its other side, then hits another tree, dragging the entire time. Freeing the sled again, his dogs pull with force over the last curve. Sebastian's sled bounces off the left-corner tree, while Sebastian himself flies over the edge, followed by his sled. The dogs manage to stay on the trail because a little sapling, perfectly located, serves as an anchor to the gang line, but the entire sled, trailer, and Sebastian are hanging off the cliff.

No time to waste, Matt Hall and I run up and form a chain of arms to pull Sebastian and his sled to safety. The instant the sled is back on the trail, the frenzied dogs take off, but Sebastian isn't ready. Caught off balance, he pinballs down the steep descent. Halfway down, he bounces off another tree; he and his sled disappear over the edge again. Sebastian sorts things out by himself this time and makes it to the bottom in one piece.

It is now my turn. Gulp. Not intimidating at all. Nope. No fear. This is the Quest: not a race for the weak-minded. I have learned through similar experiences that fear is inevitable but not insurmountable. Fear what can happen, and prepare for all outcomes. Running through all scenarios, I strategize about how to reduce risk to the dogs and to myself. Analysis calms me and helps me focus. Learning from Sebastian's experience, I take the tug lines off all but the front four dogs. This reduces the team's pulling power—I want to be in total control.

Their excitement is insane. Pulling the hook, I bounce off trees until we get stuck on the last tree on the dead man's curve overlooking the cliff to my right. I keep my hook secured to a tree so the team can't take off without me being ready. The brush brow is bent but not broken. Fifteen miles into a thousand-mile race, and the sled already has damage. I work to free the sled, then, ready, we fly down the hill. With only a few tugs attached, my speed is far less than Sebastian's. At the river bottom, we remain unhurt and in good spirits. Only 985 miles to go (see fig. 41).

This race is unique in having a thirty-six-hour mandatory rest in Dawson City. John Balzar, in his book *Yukon Alone*, remarks on Dawson: "The capital of the Klondike, with its Wild West facades and stovepipe chimneys, is recognizable from the black-and-white photographs of the Gold Rush." The Klondike Gold Rush brought more than fifty thousand prospectors into the area by 1900. We get to set up tents for dogs and mushers in the Dawson Creek campground.

I don't often, or ever, see mushers carrying tents to camp in. But last year on the Iditarod I came upon Lars Monsen, the Norwegian musher and explorer, who camps out with a tent. I pondered the scene. Why carry six more pounds to sleep an hour in comfort? Over the course of that race and the throughout the following summer, I contemplated that tent.

It takes several long minutes for body heat to radiate throughout a sleeping bag full of forty-below air. For me, I never get warm. I've tried multiple avenues to fix this. I've carried a Therm-a-Rest pad, which I blew air into, for a thermal barrier. I've put it on top of a pile of straw. My sleeping bag slid off the pad, leaving me to lie in snow and, yes, shiver. I've also tried using a Norwegian sleeping bag that acted like a thick bivy sack in which I'd put my Therm-a-Rest and my sleeping bag. While I had greater success with this approach, it weighed at least twelve pounds and still the issue of having frozen gear remained.

Enter the tent. Well-designed four-season expedition tents have a vapor barrier, which removes the warm moisture generated by breathing, perspiration, and evaporation from damp clothing that would otherwise build up in the tent and condense, keeping the inside of the tent dryer, and its occupant more comfortable.

I get one as a test, and find I get better rest when sleeping in a tent, with increased warmth versus lying on the snow. I bring a change of clothes into the tent, including a face mask, hat, socks, and inner layers. After cooking the dogs' food, I prepare my own, take three minutes to set up the tent, and throw in the Therm-a-Rest pad, sleeping bag, dry clothes, headlamp, foot and hand warmers, cooked food, two thermoses, and a pan of melted snow for hot water to make fresh coffee with.

Once inside, I throw my boots off and put them to the bottom. Staying dry, and thus warm, in sleeping bags and Arctic traveling gear is tricky. I take off my Gore-Tex outer layers and jump into the bag. Most critical is a dry face mask. Having an icy, frozen face mask made soggy by my hot breath does not make my day. I put dry gear back on because the bitter cold is dangerous. Now dry, I eat hot, delicious food while cuddled in my bag. Life is awesome. I make my coffee with the remaining melted snow water and open two hand warmers to hold close while sleeping.

I carry my five-pound Hilleberg Soulo tent from Whitehorse to Fairbanks, and I am forever in love with it. This increase in comfort is a luxury that goes a long way five hundred miles into a race.

The Quest summits don't disappoint. A storm passes through on my way over American Summit, and I freeze six fingertips during the climb up and over the summit in total-whiteout conditions. A first ascender of Denali's South Peak, and one who knows, Hudson Stuck, wrote in *Ten Thousand Miles with a Dog Sled* that "the Eagle Summit is one of the most difficult summits in Alaska. The wind blows so fiercely that sometimes for days together its passage is almost impossible." Climbing up Rosebud isn't terrible but the very steep descent through burned timber and rock is jaw-dropping.

Finishing in Fairbanks, this race is a total triumph of spirit—free of trauma, and full of the purity of a long, hard, and cold dogsled race. I do not win authenticity without a fight. By the finish of the Yukon Quest, as Rookie of the Year, there is no going back. I'm in love with the Far North and the adventures it offers (see fig. 42).

Two weeks later, we are busy preparing for the next thousand-mile race: the Iditarod.

▸NEW DREAMS

KOTZEBUE, ALASKA | 2018

You are never given a wish without also being
given the power to make it true. You may have
to work for it, however.

—RICHARD BACH

I spent the first thirty-five years of my life searching for the truth. Wilderness adventures and spiritual questing helped me find it. Searching is an ingrained habit, and for the last five years I continued to search, but I didn't know what for. Standing in your truth takes discipline and rejuvenation. It is possible to lose sight of your truth. Eager to give back to others, I jump with full attention into work and forget the basic tenants of self-care. I throw myself into coaching, family care, nonprofit work, and I forget my truth and who I am. We all find our truth in different ways. I find mine in the wilderness, meditation, and many other ways that bring me joy. Truth is the pivot point between searching and giving. To live a life of balance means standing solid in your truth. It also means knowing when we need to glide back and forth, between searching and giving, with grace.

I learn to dream again and commit to follow my dreams. I want to experience this life with a hungry passion that lay dormant after fifteen years of neglect. I want to travel to the north and south poles with a team of dogs; I want to climb the seven summits, starting with Denali; and I want to share with others that life is worth living even when it hurts.

I work to be a light in the darkness for people who are struggling to take the first step in saying yes to life every single day because of all that weighs us down. I run the 2018 Yukon Quest, only to scratch from it because of a wrist injury that renders me unable to care for my dog team. Refusing to back down, I gear up to run the 2018 Iditarod in a few weeks.

Amelia, now fifteen years old, has also learned how to dream for herself. Wanting challenge and diversity, she gets accepted to a boarding school on the East Coast—a brave girl making her own way in this big world. She inspires me daily with her courage, strength, compassion, beauty, humor, aptitude, empathy, wisdom—and I can go on forever, much to her embarrassment (see fig. 43).

Before the 2018 Iditarod, I visit Amelia, if only to hug her for a few days straight. Empty-nest syndrome does not sit well with me, so I fly out at every available opportunity. While there, I receive a call from Dave's sister-in-law, Sarah, in Ellensberg, Washington. Our young, happy-go-lucky, dimple-faced Alan shot himself in his grandparents' home, losing his battle with mental illness. Not all of us can face the overwhelming magnitude of creating new dreams. Untreated trauma can cause mental illness so severe it leaves no hope in its wake. Alan received treatment but still felt out of options.

I am there in person to tell Amelia. Her upcoming spring break allows me to take her out of school. I consider not running the 2018 Iditarod, but I want to honor Alan's memory and be strong where he couldn't. I barely remember the race, focusing so intently on keeping the team safe mile after mile. I write a eulogy while swimming through deep snow in my snowshoes.

We take an eight-hour break in Kaltag. My leader, Blondie, doesn't eat his first meal, and hours later, his breathing becomes labored. Blondie dies from hemorrhagic pneumonia ten hours after I leave Kaltag. The vets can't fly him out due to the blizzard conditions. I don't find out until I am in White Mountain, seventy-seven miles to the race finish. I ride the runners into Nome, numb and crippled by the loss of Alan and the sudden loss of my loving and fearless underdog leader.

All mushers know the deep connection found between them and their leaders. The loving dogs fill my empty heart and protect me from the raw edge of sorrow found in the indifferent solitude of the wild Arctic.

I've lost people I loved: Dave, Alan, Madi, Auntie Pam, Gramma. I've lost dogs I loved: Summit, Blondie, Flash, Rambo, Velvet, Penny, and many others as they grow old and move on to the great beyond. Each loss is as difficult as the last and tempts me to close my heart for good. Then Blondie's puppies play with me and beg for the unconditional love of my heart, and I can't hold back. Yes, to love is to risk. Scratch that. To love means you will feel pain. It is inevitable. Each time I face a choice to open up and love or to walk away, I always take that step toward being vulnerable. I owe it to those that came before me or that are no longer here to love and live fully (see fig. 44).

After completing the Iditarod, we leave the next day to attend Alan's funeral. His ashes now join the graves of Dave and Madi at our camp overlooking Kobuk Lake. Amelia and I brought him home again. No words have the power to take away the pain and emptiness all people carry from the impact of loss. I share my story to empower others to search for their way to live life to the fullest despite that pain. Find the beauty. It's epic.

►NORTHERN LIGHTS

KOBUK LAKE, ALASKA | 2018

Every end is a new beginning.

—PROVERB

On my final training run of the season, fifteen miles outside Kotzebue, I am stunned into silence by an aurora borealis light show. I ride alone—just me and my dogs in the expanse of frozen wilderness I'd dreamed about my entire life. Snow crystals glittering in the moonlight fall all around me, as if I were inside a giant snow globe.

"She saw God everywhere in the natural world and her love of nature came first, even before her children. She was a wild spirit, and she fretted being shackled, as she saw it, to the demands of two small children and poverty in city heat, away from her beloved wilderness." When I was ten, I'm sure I skipped right over this passage in *Arctic Daughter* where Jean Aspen explains her mother's fealty to the wilderness above all else. But when I read it decades later, the words made me cry. Putting myself in remote situations, where I too find God, where I need to be to exist, has exacted a high cost.

The trail brings me across Kobuk Lake, where Dave, Alan, and I had embarked on our first boat trip together in search of mammoth ivory; where I'd watched the sun rise and set every day from the windows of our camp high on the hill while cradling Madi in my arms, consumed with the bliss of new motherhood; where I'd taught Amelia how to drive a boat, run dogs, and drive a snow machine; where the dogs and I love to sing, loud and out of tune; where, with every love I've gained and lost, my heart is most at peace.

At three in the morning, an almost-full moon shines in triumph, even as a tingle of orange sunrise peeks out over the mountains to the east. Green flashes outlined in red ribbon dance in utter abandon across the deep black sky. The lights seem to be hanging so low in the atmosphere I can almost touch them. I watch in awe. I look forward to describing tonight to Amelia, who shares my wonderment at the night sky.

All my life I have chased the northern lights, which always provide the brightest illumination during the deepest, darkest night. Tonight I say a prayer of thanks for the three-minute display that ends without warning, just as it began, filling my heart with gratitude as I realize that my daughter, now a courageous, independent young woman, will one day soon be hungrily chasing down her own northern lights. Then, I continue mushing toward home.

ACKNOWLEDGMENTS

To all those on the other side of the door:

Of course, Mom and Dad; my stepdad, John, and stepmom, Linda; J.T. Gleason; Cassie Thill; Cindy Foster; Katie Nordahl; Judith Ragir; Cheryl Knight; Autcha Kameroff and Ruth-Ann Zent; Dickie and Sandra Moto; Tracey and Chuck Schaeffer; Eric Smith; Bill and Sue Rimer; The Keith Family; all of Team Baker; John Baker; and last but not least, Amelia Keith.

Then there are those who helped turn this book from concept to reality:

Matt Crossman, whose journalistic talents first put my truth on paper; Katie Orlinsky, who can make one photo speak louder than a book; Jonathan Lyons of Curtis Brown LTD, for believing in me; Vikki Warner of Blackstone Publishing, for believing in my story; Alenka Linaschke of Blackstone Publishing, for her stunning designs; Jessica DuLong, for helping me find my voice; Michael Krohn and Peggy Hageman, for making sure that voice was grammatical;

And all the others along the way whose actions, small and large, kept me searching for the next stake.